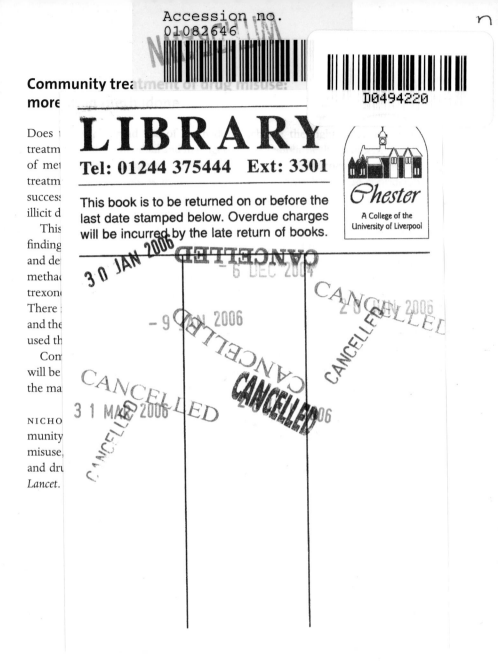

**Community tre**
**more**

Does
treatm
of met
treatm
success
illicit d
    This
finding
and de
methad
trexone
There
and the
used th
    Com
will be
the ma

NICHO
munity
misuse,
and dru
Lancet.

# Community treatment of drug misuse:
## more than methadone

NICHOLAS SEIVEWRIGHT

Consultant Psychiatrist in Substance Misuse, Community Health Sheffield NHS Trust

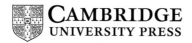

CAMBRIDGE
UNIVERSITY PRESS

PUBLISHED BY THE PRESS SYNDICATE OF THE UNIVERSITY OF CAMBRIDGE
The Pitt Building, Trumpington Street, Cambridge, United Kingdom

CAMBRIDGE UNIVERSITY PRESS
The Edinburgh Building, Cambridge CB2 2RU, UK
40 West 20th Street, New York, NY 10011–4211, USA
477 Williamstown Road, Port Melbourne, VIC 3207, Australia
Ruiz de Alarcón 13,28014 Madrid, Spain
Dock House, The waterfront, Cape Town 8001, South Africa

http://www.cambridge.org

First published 2000
Reprinted 2000, 2001

Printed in the United Kingdom at the University Press, Cambridge

Typeset in Dante MT 11/13pt [VN]

A catalogue record for this book is available from the British Library

Library of Congress Cataloguing in Publication data

0 521 59091 4 hardback
0 521 66562 0 paperback

Every effort has been made in preparing this book to provide accurate and up-to-date information which is in accord with accepted standards and practice at the time of publication. Nevertheless, the authors, editors and publisher can make no warranties that the information contained herein is totally free from error, not least because standards are constantly changing through research and regulation. The authors, editors and publisher therefore disclaim all liability for direct or consequential damages resulting from the use of material contained in this book. Readers are strongly advised to pay careful attention to information provided by the manufacturer of any drugs or equipment that they plan to use.

# Contents

## Part II Providing clinical services

# Foreword

Dr Seivewright has produced an excellent handbook on the community treatment of drug misuse. Essentially, his book is a workshop manual for the practitioner faced with any one of the many challenges which may confront the medical or nonmedical drug worker in the UK. Just as a car workshop manual can guide both the novice and the more experienced mechanic through tasks ranging from the change of a lightbulb through to a complete engine re-fit, so Dr Seivewright's book can guide the novice or experienced drug worker through tasks as varied as dose assessment to the organization of integrated service provision across primary and secondary care. Dr Seivewright is excellently well suited to prepare this book, bringing, on the one hand, the experience and wisdom of a battle-scarred clinician who has already worked for many years in charge of drug services in the UK and, on the other hand, the discipline and critical scrutiny of the academic in his search and analysis of the available international evidence for the treatments he describes.

*More than Methadone.* As the sub-title of the book indicates, the challenge and responsibility of better community treatment of drug misuse involves much more than methadone. Whilst parts of the book deal with ways of optimizing methadone treatment itself, other important sections deal with other aspects of a comprehensive holistic approach to care of the heterogeneous population who comprise the treatment population of today's drug services. When methadone is prescribed, there are many different ways in which the drug may be used to assist recovery. Even within a particular treatment modality such as methadone maintenance, the treatment philosophy which the clinician and the patient/client espouse will vary greatly from one country to another, and also from one agency to the next – consider, for example, the sharply different ways in which methadone is being employed in either the 'medical model' or the 'substitution model' explored by Dr Seivewright on page 22 and thereafter. And how should one bear in mind the complicating factor of concurrent use of other drugs – either as an additional complicating aspect of the original presenting problem, or as one of the necessary ongoing outcome measures during the course of treatment. There is then the enormously important consideration of the context within which methadone might be prescribed. The drug may be the same, but there is a world of difference between a well managed clinic and the casual or careless prescribing of a week's supply of methadone by the uninterested GP or hospital doctor who just wants to get the patient out of the consulting room – same drug, but a million miles away from the objective and the approach that should be seen in the well organized service. And, at a very literal level, there is now more than methadone. Until recently methadone was the only medication with a product licence for the treatment of the active opiate addict. Like an artist moving from black and white to colour, today's clinician now has different colours from which to choose. In addition to methadone, a substantial evidence base has been established in the UK around use of lofexidine for opiate detoxification, to which have recently been added buprenorphine for use as a new opiate maintenance pharmacotherapy and LAAM, the long acting pro-drug methadone analogue (both the latter two drugs having been investigated extensively in the US but still currently in their infancy within the UK). Compared with the dark days of yesteryear, the clinician of today is spoilt for choice with regard to selection of specific pharmacotherapy.

Dr Seivewright's book will guide the reader safely around the different possible choices so as to make optimal use of *Community Treatment of Drug Misuse.*

JOHN STRANG
*Professor and Director*
*National Addiction Centre*
*London, UK*

# Preface and acknowledgements

When I was asked to write a book on drug misuse treatment, I felt that he most important objective was to make it true to life. Treatment of this group can be highly problematic, and to say that things often do not go according to plan is a great understatement. Many doctors and other clinicians are reluctant to be involved, deterred by the behavioural problems, apparent lack of impact of treatments, and other obvious difficulties. The last thing anyone needs is a book which implies that the various treatments can be selected and applied in a simple manner, with ordinary compliance just as in any other condition.

Drug misusers, especially of long standing, tend to have stronger views on their problem than people who have other disorders. They cannot be expected to be neutral about whether they are to receive methadone, whether treatment starts immediately or next month, what dosage of various medications they are to have or, indeed, whether they are likely to go to prison or not. The nature of the condition means that there will be much direct investment in these things, and clinicians are not on the whole well suited to drug misuse if they object to being told how to do their job now and again. Patients may attempt to 'misuse' services – and certainly medications – as they do drugs, and any good instruction must acknowledge these kinds of difficulties, and their influence on treatment.

As well as wanting to give the book a sufficiently practical orientation, there were other aspects which appeared important. I was glad that it was to be in a series which concentrates on the social dimension, since social aspects are of huge relevance in drug misuse. In psychiatric practice I have long been aware that aspects such as personality, lifestyle and subculture are typically far bigger determinants of progress than the minutiae of mental state symptoms, and dealing with drug problems especially bears this out. The psychiatry involved in this work is of a very particular type, and a sensitivity to social considerations is vital. I have described the main treatment, methadone, in Chapter 1 as being a medical treatment for social reasons, and in our specialty we are well used to measuring outcomes predominantly in the social arena.

The theme of there being more to treatment than methadone does not derive from any fundamental reservations about substitution treatment, as any pragmatic clinician should acknowledge that this is essential to have, if only because of general relapse rates. The point is rather that in recent years we have been so dominated by methadone that we have neglected other areas. With 'low-threshold' methadone prescribing having been recommended to try to stem the HIV epidemic, huge numbers have ended up on the treatment, in addition to the more established maintenance candidates. As well as wondering how long such treatment is justified, many workers in drug services are concerned that the needs of other users are simply not being met. Young and early-stage heroin users require detoxification treatments, but time must be available for this relatively intensive work. Those who are struggling in their attempts to stay off opiates may only get much attention if methadone becomes indicated. Users of ecstasy, amphetamines, crack cocaine and other drugs barely get a look in. Even with the maintenance candidates, is methadone the best drug? What are the advantages of buprenorphine or LAAM? Why is it said so consistently by some that it would be better to prescribe diamorphine, and that methadone is more toxic, addictive and dangerous? While acknowledging the place of methadone, this book also examines the evidence for a wide range of treatments across the various forms of drug misuse, to help us attempt to offer more comprehensive and equitable services.

There are many commonalities within drug misuse across the world, and this book deliberately adopts an international perspective. There are also many important differences, with some of the most interesting relating to differing treatment policies, and examples of these are explored in several sections. To explain where I am 'coming from', both literally and figuratively, and to acknowledge the help of many people along the way, I will briefly recount my involvement in this specialty.

In 1982, my very first trainee job in psychiatry was in Nottingham with Professor Peter Tyrer, who asked me to write this book. I am extremely grateful for the invitation, and even more so for the help and guidance he has given me over all the intervening years. I can only assume he spotted my interest in personality, and therefore personality disorder, as he has involved me in many projects on this subject, and others to do with neurotic disorder, psychiatric services and psycho-pharmacology. As well as being my academic mentor, he instilled in me the principles of community psychiatry, since that first posting and the later research settings were modelled along those lines, and I have professionally grown up with that way of working. My wife Helen, who is a general practitioner and genitourinary physician with an interest in psychiatry, is involved with some of our projects, and Peter has been equally supportive towards her.

As part of the Nottingham rotational training scheme, two years after starting I had a posting at the Nottingham regional addiction unit, with Dr Philip McLean. This was my first experience in drug and alcohol treatment, and I must have enjoyed it, as I have been in it ever since! I did sessional attachments throughout the research fellowship, and as part of all my other postings. This was mainstream clinical experience in a very well established service, and I found that the subject interested me more than any other subspecialty. I therefore have another great debt of gratitude to Dr McLean, who taught me all the basics about the addictions and much more – I think the clinical realism comes from him.

One day in 1988 Dr McLean returned from a visit to inspect the services in Manchester, to say that there was a vacancy as consultant at the Regional Drug Dependence Service there. This was the unit in Prestwich from which Professor John Strang directed the setting up of 19 community drug teams in the surrounding areas, an impressive network which has, through the literature, given us much knowledge about this model of working. With Professor Strang having returned to London, and following a tenure of the post by Dr Chris Fisher, I was appointed to that job and stayed in Manchester for an extremely interesting and formative six years. Patients who required referral to the regional service from the community drug teams were often severely dependent, and it was there that I gained most experience of seeing individuals who were incapable of adjusting to methadone treatment. We had many patients on injectable drugs, and diamorphine and other alternatives were required in some cases. Most of these maintenance patients were not only heavily dependent on opiates but habitually used other drugs, and it was all too apparent that the methadone mixture often cannot serve the needs of such individuals. Not all the patients I saw were of this type as I also did sessions at two of the community drug teams, with a more 'normal' kind of caseload. The experience was therefore very broad, and I was pleased to play a part in helping the service become fully active again after a period with no one in post.

In due course in Manchester I was appointed to a Senior Lecturer position in drug dependence, and I am grateful for the guidance in my University work from Professors David Goldberg, Bill Deakin and Francis Creed. I was therefore only half-time in direct clinical work, and the person most responsible for building up the Manchester service (now called Drugs North West), was my colleague Dr John Merrill, who came one year after me. He has a great commitment to the service and to the field of drug misuse, and with three further consultants now there, Manchester is rightly regarded as one of the leading specialist centres in the UK. I also benefitted during my time there from the expertise of Dr Michael Donmall, an authority on drug misuse epidemiology, whose academic unit was linked with our clinical service, and we have since collaborated on research in cocaine misuse.

My family and I decided that we wished to move back to Nottinghamshire, and to enable this I secured my present job as consultant in Sheffield. This can definitely be called a challenge, as this city of over half a million people has never had an established clinical service for substance misuse treatment. I am grateful to those who had some sessional involvement before I came, particularly Professors Alec Jenner and Philip Seager, and then (in addition to other full-time jobs!) Mr Peter Pratt, Director of Pharmacy and service director, and Dr Andrew MacNeill, Medical Director of the Trust. Peter continues highly effectively as service director, and I have nothing but admiration for the Substance Misuse Team working to establish our presence in the city: Phil Clay, Fran Roman, Kevin Murphy, Giz Sangha, Karen Roach, Sarah Crookes, Michelle Horspool, Kath Barnes and Roger Marshall, and Nik Howes who liaises with us from the Rockingham Drug Project. I am particularly impressed by the work of Sean Meehan, Team Leader, who literally leads by professional example. I have also been grateful for the help of Dr Charlie McMahon, our previous senior trainee who has since moved to become consultant in addictions in Paisley, Scotland, Dr Roger Smith, highly experienced general practitioner and clinical assistant in Sheffield, and Dr Chris Sudell, who has recently started with us in Nottinghamshire.

I have described in the book some of the work of the two services in which I am employed. Whereas most of the patients whom I see personally in Sheffield are in the substitution treatment clinics, in North Nottinghamshire I have for three years been the only doctor with the service, and so I see a broader range, including many detoxification candidates. This has been particularly instructive, as the services in Nottingham, Manchester and Sheffield have all been, to varying degrees and for different reasons, inclined towards treating more severe patients. My views on treatment have been strongly influenced by the extremely impressive work that is done in the North Nottinghamshire service, and the sections in the book on detoxification and relapse prevention, drug counselling, and treatment of nonopiate misusers in particular owe much to discussions and joint working with the individual team members. They are: Paul Sales (service coordinator), Donnamarie Donnelly, Majella Kenny, Sarah Peat, Nick Coombs, Cathy Symes, Matt Downing, Jonathan Law and Paul Berry. Although mildly dependent heroin users present to most services, it takes a skilled and very systematic approach to consistently see such users successfully through detoxification, and it is clear to me that this service enables many individuals to become drug free who would, at best, be languishing on methadone if their contact was elsewhere.

There are many other clinical colleagues from the UK and other countries who have taught me much about drug misuse treatment. They are far too numerous to mention, but in offering a general thank you, I will single out Professor John Strang and Drs Michael Farrell, Duncan Raistrick, Philip Fleming, Judy Myles and Colin Brewer, who have all specifically advised me on subjects included here. I was also extremely interested to have several discussions with Dr Alex Wodak and Professor Greg Whelan when I was kindly invited to give a short series of lectures in Australia in 1995, and colleagues in Europe, notably including Dr Henrik Rindom in Copenhagen, and in the USA, have been similarly helpful. Another great opportunity was to coedit and contribute to an international series on addictions for *The Lancet*, and I am grateful for that to the editors of the journal, particularly Ms Pia Pini, and to my coeditor, Dr Judy Greenwood. A short review of current issues in treatment (Seivewright & Greenwood 1996) provided the basis for some of the ideas in this book. Even having had all these many positive influences, however, there will be deficiencies in the personal view which this book inevitably partly represents, and I bear full responsibility for any of those.

Most directly, I thank the two colleagues without whom the book simply could not have been written: Amy Haddon, my secretary, who typed many drafts and did much associated work while keeping up with the usual National Health Service commitments, and Victor Thompson, research assistant, who undertook the literature searches in an expert manner. Personally, I am grateful in the extreme to my wife, Helen, and our children, Paula and Richard, for their forbearance during my work on the project.

The final note about the book concerns the case histories, which I feel are an important aspect. To preserve anonymity these are composite histories, each containing elements from more than one case, but they intentionally illustrate the common problems – and successes – which typically emerge in real clinical practice, which straightforward accounts of treatments cannot always convey.

NICHOLAS SEIVEWRIGHT

# Introduction: community treatment in context

In providing clinical treatment for drug misuse we play one part in addressing a problem which is among the most serious facing modern society. The use of illicit drugs has escalated hugely in recent years in many countries across the world, with wider causes which are beyond our control as, indeed, are any overall solutions. Most of the trends which have led to such high rates of drug misuse show no signs of abating, and political arguments rage as to the relative merits of differing social policies and approaches to drug legislation. Within this, as clinicians we have a specific prime responsibility to treat individuals who present with identifiable drug problems, plus an additional implicit role in helping those affected by such use, and we must be able to fulfil these as successfully as possible, as part of the much bigger picture. This requires an informed knowledge of all the approaches which can best help individuals to stop taking drugs or to reduce their usage in their various personal situations, and can limit the associated problems in homes, families, and communities.

This book aims to help in that task by reviewing practically the treatments which are indicated across a broad range of clinical situations. In recent times the treatment scene internationally has been dominated by methadone, the so-called 'heroin substitute' which can enable users to avoid the various consequences of taking illicit drugs. The substitution approach is inherently controversial, in that it necessarily replaces one drug of addiction with another and has no real equivalent in the way we manage other dependencies, but it is undoubtedly here to stay, with strong evidence for general effectiveness in severely dependent individuals. With ever-broader usage, however, including the attempts to stem the HIV epidemic, the problems and limitations of methadone have become increasingly apparent, and the possible alternatives which may be safer or less addictive, or offer other clinical advantages, are reviewed here. There is also a more general concern among workers in services that the emphasis on opioid maintenance treatment completely skews presentation rates so that, unless positive steps are taken, little attention is paid to users of nonopiate drugs or to less dependent individuals. I have

1

included a review of treatments for misuse of the wider range of drugs, while at the heart of the book is an account of the work we do in helping users achieve detoxification from heroin and other opiates. Candidates for detoxification treatments rather than maintenance methadone can only increase as heroin becomes widely available and more and more young people begin using it; services need to target such individuals, to offer treatment before addiction becomes established. The way in which we deploy our own community services is described, and there are discussions of the important aspects of practical provision for various clinical groups. Our services have a strong community psychiatric orientation, which includes the principle of working with primary care physicians wherever possible, and many of the treatments which are described in the book are also applicable in that setting.

The number one priority in writing the chapters which follow has been to examine *realistically* the treatments we use in day-to-day practice, with reference to many of the problems which can occur in managing this often difficult population. In terms of an additional theoretical perspective, undoubtedly the social aspects of drug misuse are those which are particularly emphasized. As a clinician in this field it is impossible not to be struck by the social considerations at virtually every turn – in the associated problems of individuals, characteristic subcultural aspects in different types of usage, social origins of drug use, social consequences, and in the nature of many of the benefits of treatment. This dimension of the drug misuse phenomenon will be a recurring theme throughout the book, so that, for instance, the next chapter recognizes that the social effects of methadone treatment are more striking than any other kind, raising fundamental questions about the nature and purposes of this treatment approach.

This introductory chapter takes one step back from the treatment situation, to examine the social background against which drug misuse is often set, some of the aetiological factors, and the place which clinical treatment occupies in the wider scheme of things. It is by way of a brief and fairly subjective overview, before the treatment approaches are examined in greater detail, in various international contexts. In our own services we use inpatient or residential options only very rarely, and so they are summarized at the end of the chapter, with some additional consideration where relevant in later chapters.

# Drug misuse as a social problem

The use of various substances has very different meanings in different cultures and countries (Westermeyer 1995). In addition, attitudes to drugs do not remain static, but change over time, as we are witnessing at present in relation to cannabis. In general, however, in blunt behavioural terms, it may be said that the taking of any drug which is currently illegal, whatever we may think of the legislature, represents a more 'deviant' behaviour than taking a drug which is legal, however harmful that drug may in fact be. In many countries, clinically significant illicit drug use often arises in the context of other broadly antisocial activities, being associated in the same geographical areas and, to varying degrees, in the same individuals. Concentrations of drug misuse occur in environments with high levels of school truancy, gang activities and various types of crime, and a history of these may be found in those presenting for drug treatment. In such situations, even when a genetic theory of substance misuse is tempting, for instance if a parent has been a heavy drinker, lifestyle factors can seem just as important, with each generation using the available substances as part of a general behavioural and social pattern. The evidence for actual familial transmission in illicit drug abuse has been reviewed by Ripple & Luthar (1996), while we may speculate that the social influences may be even stronger in those outside treatment, for whom drug use may be effectively a recreational activity.

In cities and towns particularly, the rates of drug use and other antisocial problems appear to increase steadily, with ever-younger individuals involved. The social causes are no doubt similar to those in personality disorder which have been examined by Paris (1996a) in an earlier volume in this series: these include family breakdown, parental psychopathology, weakening of the effect of authority systems, and social disintegration in communities, in which there are reduced constraints on antisocial behaviour. With the demonstrations of increased prevalence of drug use, including school surveys, the activity can be said to be becoming more normative. In such circumstances the levels of associated problems and psychopathology among those who use drugs may be expected to reduce, but this has so far not been demonstrated, and it can equally be claimed that in countries where there is an overall rise in drug misuse, this is partly an indicator of generally increasing social problems.

There is clearly a big difference between the occasional use of cannabis and dependence on 'hard' drugs in the various social aspects, including the context of usage and, especially, the social consequences. Much of the widespread recreational drug use may produce no discernible social problems, with the exception of the consequences of legal sanctions if caught. However, as usage progresses, and in a kind of gradient across the range of drugs, social consequences may include family and relationship problems, isolation from those except other drug users, reduced job prospects, debt, crime and adverse effects on child care (Kolar et al. 1994). The relationship with crime is not a straightforward one, and even acquisitive crime by drug users cannot simply be explained by funding expensive drug habits. Increasingly those involved in crime or antisocial behaviours will tend to use illicit drugs as a lifestyle feature, just as they tend to smoke. Whatever the connections, the criminal justice system can be a good place to engage drug users to offer advice and treatment, and within Europe, the Netherlands has led the way in providing arrest referral schemes (Wolters 1995).

With such strong social factors operating, many clinicians outside drug misuse treatment take some persuading that the condition significantly represents a clinical one at all, as opposed to a problem requiring social solutions. However, the general syndrome of dependence has strong psychological elements and, as we shall see, can be effectively addressed in drug counselling, provided an assertive enough clinical approach is adopted. Psychiatrists have a definite role because of the predominance of associated psychiatric problems, albeit usually the partly socially defined ones of conduct and personality disorders, and there is the whole area of medical management of complications. Most basically, drugs are psychoactive substances and the more that drug dependence progresses, the more clinical its treatment becomes. Within this, there is no doubt that social benefits are necessarily part of the aim of treatment, and the exploration of the unusual position of providing pharmacological treatments directly to achieve such outcomes begins in the next chapter.

## Risk factors for drug misuse

Social and psychiatric research have both made substantial contributions on the subject of the aetiology of drug misuse. An unfortunate aspect of the literature is that there is little overlap between the disciplines, so that subjects such as unemployment or social disadvantage on the one hand, and personality or psychopathology on the other, tend to be discussed without much acknowledgement of areas of overlap. Table 1 indicates some of the risk factors for drug misuse, and the main contention here is that the personal and social factors are importantly interlinked.

Table 1. *Related risk factors for drug misuse*

| Personal | Social |
| --- | --- |
| Disrupted family of origin | Deprivation |
| Childhood trauma | Poor environment |
| Abuse | Frequent adverse life events |
| Adolescent conduct disorder | Relationship problems |
| Educational difficulties | Unemployment |
| Antisocial personality disorder | Lack of social opportunities |

Within the personal factors, clearly family disruption, trauma and physical or sexual abuse can all predispose to conduct disorder in adolescence and personality disorder in adulthood (Paris 1996b). Links between such factors and adolescent substance misuse have been consistently found (Patton 1995), while the associations between established personality disorder and drug misuse are among the strongest in the clinical literature (Seivewright & Daly 1997). In terms of interconnections, the range of background problems can produce difficulties in forming and sustaining relationships, and personality disorder is associated with high rates of ongoing adverse life events, which are usually seen as social factors (Poulton & Andrews 1992). Personal factors may also lead to unemployment, as may educational difficulties, which predispose to drug use partly through disengagement from the school system. Lone parenthood is associated with substance misuse in adolescent children (Miller 1997), but such parents are at increased risk of both psychopathology and disadvantage in housing.

A short review of the demonstrated relationships between social deprivation and drug use has been provided by Pearson (1996). He notes not only the correlations with unemployment, the dispiriting effects of which are usually all too obvious in practice, but also the 'local informal economies of crime and hustling which thrive in areas lacking opportunities for involvement in the formal economy'. As if the risk factors for drug misuse were not related enough, he also describes the melting pot effect of problem housing estates. Tenants largely comprise those who cannot obtain anywhere preferable, including the previously homeless, teenagers in their first accommodation, women escaping domestic violence, and the elderly poor. If drug misusers are also added, or arrive through squatting, drug use can spread rapidly in fertile ground. This scenario, compounded by a lack of other social opportunities, is very familiar to those of us providing services in large cities.

## The role of treatment

Given the complex nature of the phenomenon which comprises the various forms of drug misuse, what is the role of treatment, and who should receive it? Drug services certainly need to concentrate their efforts on providing treatments which are effective, and the later chapters are aimed at shedding light on that aspect. Even the concept of effectiveness is not straightforward, however, and in our multi-faceted subject we must avoid being trapped into too narrow a concept of 'evidence-based practice'. Giving methadone is a fundamentally different type of treatment to most others offered in drug misuse and, not surprisingly, has the strongest supporting evidence by far, but it is wrong to provide that to the virtual exclusion of other approaches which may be useful in many cases. The particular problems of adhering to evidence-based practice in drug misuse are discussed in the Epilogue, and the indications for the various respective treatment methods in the intervening chapters, but the question of who it is suitable to attempt to treat at all bears some examination here.

The two simplest answers to the question of who to treat are: those who want to be treated, and/or those who have an established problem of definite dependence. (The management of medical and psychiatric complications can be seen as a separate issue, although there is much overlap in practice, as will be discussed.) Such selection has become somewhat diluted in recent years, notably following the involvement of drug users in the HIV epidemic, and consequent initiatives such as injecting equipment provision, harm reduction advice for those who continue to use drugs, and generally more accessible treatment (see Chapter 7). Also, in terms of motivating factors, there are many probation-linked schemes for those who may not otherwise have sought treatment, but who comply as an alternative to custody. While the need for these various approaches is undeniable, the broadening of acceptance criteria poses a number of problems which should be acknowledged.

First, the number of referrals can rapidly become quite unmanageable. Although it is impossible to know the true prevalence of drug misuse for any area, in a city of 600 000 people such as Sheffield the number using opiates, cocaine or large amounts of amphetamines is probably in the order of 10 000. Even the best-established treatment service would have problems coping with one-tenth of that number, and resources are simply never going to be available to cater for the full demand. Secondly, there may be a distinct lack of impact if treatment is offered uncritically to those in whom drug use is basically a symptom of multiple social problems, as discussed above. Although the presence of other problems is definitely no bar to treatment, and indeed looking at drug use can be a 'way in' to offering consistent professional help with various general benefits, the role of drug treatment in such circumstances must not be overplayed. Thirdly, with a wide variety of types of drug misuser presenting from different referral sources, prioritization can be extremely problematic, especially if some emphasis on what may be broadly termed motivation is to be retained.

In many ways it is useful to have drug services operating on two different levels. Basic facilities such as injecting equipment provision, information, advice on a drop-in basis, and supportive counselling should be made widely available, with as few barriers as possible. There is then a need for a *clinical* treatment service, to provide the range of specific behavioural interventions and pharmacological treatments for suitable individuals, with some limitation in access inevitable. In community-based treatment services it is usually still a guiding principle to offer treatment to as many users as possible, and the operation in this way of our own services and of community drug teams in general is discussed further in Chapter 5.

The overall response to drug problems includes prevention, education, treatment and enforcement. To debate the appropriate relative contribution of these elements is beyond the scope of this brief discussion, but it is clear that all organizations involved with drug misuse largely fail to keep pace with the rising rates of the problem, or to make significant impressions on the drugs scene in general. Nonenforcement prevention initiatives have tended to drift towards 'secondary' prevention, basically a form of harm reduction, in effect accepting ongoing drug use. The effects of drugs education are largely unproven, but at the same time those who know at first hand the difficulty of managing established cases of drug misuse should accept that, if possible, prevention is better than cure. Meanwhile the criminal justice systems in many countries simply do not have the capacity to deal with all the drug offenders, and sentencing is often light across the range of drugs. The changing role of enforcement has been discussed by Hellawell (1995), who became the UK's first antidrugs coordinator ('drug czar'), while an important point which affects the balance between the various systems is that not all forms of drug misuse are equally amenable to treatment. As we shall see, nearly all the established specific clinical interventions are for opiate misuse, including the option of methadone which has no parallel in other drug problems. The more challenging nature of managing nonopiate misuse is often not appreciated by other agencies, and drug services need to advise others realistically about the potency of clinical approaches, in situations such as diversion from court.

In the south of England, Robson & Bruce (1997) compared 'visible' and 'invisible' users of amphetamine, cocaine and heroin, postulating that these were two distinct populations. The invisible group, i.e. unknown to drug services, mostly expressed little or no concern about their drug use and no wish for help or advice. They were mainly stimulant users, and less likely to inject or, if they did, to share equipment. They had lower scores on a formal dependence rating and were less likely to use daily. The visible group, who had had contact with treatment services, were predominantly opiate users, using daily. Although the populations cannot be completely separate, as any user in contact for the first time self-evidently changes from one group to the other, the study reinforced the observations that not all drug users wish to have treatment, and that services mainly treat opiate users. The authors conclude that 'purchasers and providers with limited resources should concentrate on improving the range and quality of services for users already in contact rather than attempting to uncover invisible populations'.

## Inpatient and residential treatment

Of our own services, in North Nottinghamshire we have no inpatient facility, whilst in Sheffield we have five beds for substance misuse on one of the psychiatric wards, which we use mainly for alcohol patients. This is partly historical: North Nottinghamshire used to be subsumed under the Nottingham regional addiction service which has a large specialist in-patient unit, before becoming a separate service for administrative reasons, whilst in Sheffield there has not been a firmly established clinical service until recently. However, we also consider the strong emphasis on community treatment a desirable position, as we only see inpatient treatment being indicated for an extremely small proportion of drug misusers. We can refer to the Nottingham unit in such cases or use our own limited facility in Sheffield, while as with any other drug service in the UK there can be access to any of the range of independent residential rehabilitation centres. The main aspects of these two types of treatment setting are summarized below.

## Inpatient treatment

This may be used for detoxification from one or more drugs, management of medical and psychiatric complications, initiating substitution treatments in particularly problematic cases, or various forms of respite. For detoxification it seems clear that a specialist unit for drug misusers is usually a preferable setting to a general ward. Apart from the difficulties which drug misusers and general psychiatric patients may have in getting on with each other, staff need to be well versed in matters such as obtaining daily urine samples and restricting visitors and time off the unit, and in various manipulations which are characteristic in such admissions. There need to be treatment contracts, and on a specialized unit there can be a therapy programme designed for drug users, rather than attempts to fit in with more general options. At worst, some nonspecialized staff have little sympathy for withdrawal discomfort, which can produce an angry response from drug users. In the UK, inpatient drug programmes are usually pragmatically based, with keyworker sessions and some group work focusing on areas such as coping with withdrawal, anxiety management, relapse prevention and drug-free lifestyles. There may be input from Narcotics Anonymous, while some units, particularly in the private sector, are based exclusively on the 12-step approach (Cook 1988). This has the advantage of being a very assertive and unequivocal method but, in our populations, drug misusers tend to accept it less well than alcohol misusers; indeed, combining both groups can itself sometimes be problematic.

The question of whether treatment in a specialist unit is more successful than on a general psychiatric ward was tested in a randomized trial by Strang et al. (1997). The specialist unit appeared more acceptable, with almost a quarter of those who were randomized to the general ward failing to accept that allocation, and fewer subsequently presenting for admission there than at the unit. Completion rates were also higher in the specialist setting although, importantly, that group received methadone whereas patients on the general ward had clonidine only. During seven-month follow-up, significantly more patients from the specialist unit had remained drug-free than from the general ward.

Some of the most interesting options in opiate withdrawal are those that achieve detoxification quicker than a standard methadone withdrawal. These include the precipitation of withdrawal by opiate antagonists (e.g. Merrill & Marshall 1997) and even detoxification under general anaesthesia, and the various methods of inpatient opiate detoxification are discussed further in Chapter 3. The clonidine analogue, lofexidine, is commonly used in the UK, which we use as our main method of quick community detoxification from heroin (see Chapter 3).

### Residential rehabilitation

This is a lengthy treatment, with rehabilitation centres often taking clients for 6–12 months or more for residential treatment. Some use 12-step methods (Cook 1988), while some are run by religious organizations or according to a strong 'concept' theme. In Sheffield we have one of the Phoenix House centres which are established internationally. Often, residential centres are away from main centres of population and, indeed, addicts are usually advised to go to one in another area, to consolidate their break from their drug-using scene.

Some centres provide a short detoxification, or this may be done just before going in. Often this is requested as an inpatient, since those users felt that to require residential rehabilitation may also be considered too dependent to complete reliably a detoxification in the community. Many inpatient services therefore prioritize individuals who have a rehabilitation place waiting. The group and individual therapy in rehabilitation centres typically concentrates not only on personal issues, but on making fundamental lifestyle changes (Lewis et al. 1993). Very assertive tactics may be brought to bear to counter the behaviours that are seen as characteristic, such as deception and exploitation. The treatment is demanding, but is intended to be somewhat more curative than clinical approaches are generally considered to be. Selection is very important, as many users are unable to truly make a commitment to a long-term residential treatment of this nature. Phoenix House in Sheffield operates a family unit, where drug misusers who are parents can have residential treatment with their children staying with them.

### General observations

Inpatient hospital treatment and residential rehabilitation are very different in character, and in average length of stay. It is very useful to have both available as options for selected cases, but clearly they cannot be used at all routinely, because of sheer numbers of drug users presenting, and the strong preference which most have for being treated at home.

Some general observations may be made, which to varying extents apply to both settings. The assessment of cases for possible admission to an inpatient or residential unit should preferably involve a member of staff from the unit, to enable the most accurate briefing about treatment conditions, rules and regulations. This is especially important since, as with alcohol cases, there is something of a received wisdom that inpatient detoxification is indicated for those individuals who have too many adverse prognostic features to be successful at detoxification as an outpatient, such as heavy usage, multiple drugs, long history, personality disorder, and poor social situation. In practice, not only are such individuals also the least likely to complete detoxification successfully as an inpatient, but they are often especially unable to tolerate the constraints of a hospital setting. Discharges for self-medication or behavioural disturbances are common, and in general a high degree of proficiency is required in these settings, and in assessment procedures, to avoid what may be termed a 'severity paradox', in which success is positively unlikely in those who are particularly considered to require the approach.

Exactly what constitutes 'success' is contentious in any drug misuse treatment, but one point is brought into particularly sharp focus in relation to the inpatient and residential options. This is the question of success at detoxification – do we mean just that, or are we by implication taking into account whether an individual actually stays off drugs afterwards? The purist view is well stated by Wodak (1994): '[Detoxification] should be considered successful if safe and comfortable withdrawal has been achieved, whether or not this is followed by a permanent state of abstinence. The ultimate achievement of abstinence, if that should happen, should be regarded as a bonus . . . detoxification should therefore be regarded as very different from other forms of treatment, and possibly should not even be considered to be a form of treatment.' In a review of the effectiveness of detoxification, Mattick & Hall (1996) say something similar: 'Many countries adopt services that seem to be based on the belief that detoxification can bring about lasting changes in drug use, despite evidence to the contrary. Detoxification is more appropriately regarded as a process that aims to achieve a safe and humane withdrawal from a drug of dependence. This is a worthwhile aim in itself.' While the clear separation of the elements of detoxification and subsequent relapse prevention is indeed an important clinical principle, many observers, including those who fund treatments, may legitimately expect that labour- and cost-intensive residential options should have a more lasting impact, to be justified. To take extremes, the situation of someone relapsing into heroin use one week after a short course of medication as an outpatient is less unfortunate than someone relapsing one week after 18 months of intensive residential therapy and, in fairness, the long-term rehabilitation centres generally accept that higher 'obligation'. As clinicians we must use the treatment methods that appear appropriate in each case, but in our services, as in many others, we acknowledge that we strongly favour community treatment, mainly on the grounds of patient preference, but also to maximize the number of individuals who can receive treatment from limited resources.

The strongest traditions of inpatient detoxification relate mainly to alcohol misuse, in which the withdrawal syndrome is inherently more dangerous than that from opiates, and the avoidance of withdrawal complications in standard treatment may be the prime consideration in selecting admission. (In drug misuse, as we shall see in subsequent chapters, indications for admission increasingly relate to new developments, such as the experimental techniques for rapid detoxification from opiates, or severe clinical states produced by crack cocaine.) The drug misuse treatment scene is very different from that in alcohol in many ways, but most notably because of the acceptance of a substitution treatment approach in the form of methadone, and this produces another difficulty in relation to inpatient and residential treatment. Again as will be discussed in detail, methadone maintenance has been strongly encouraged on harm reduction grounds since the threat of HIV among drug misusers, and clinicians have become nervous of opiate users being in difficulties without this medication. When a methadone patient is admitted for detoxification, it is therefore very difficult to strike the right balance as to how readily methadone should be made available to them again if they run into problems. If it is virtually guaranteed that they can have their methadone back should they prove unable to cope with the detoxification, that can have a major demotivating effect, while if that safety net is not there, users who might be able to detoxify will be deterred. Of course, this difficulty also applies to community detoxifications from methadone, but in the case of costly inpatient treatment the implications of aborting a detoxification to re-establish methadone are magnified.

The particular problems of inpatient care and long-term residential rehabilitation for drug misusers are best addressed by those with a substantial commitment to such treatment, including services with specialist inpatient units for this group (Strang et al. 1997). Such units can offer a range of detoxification techniques and variable periods in which rehabilitation needs are examined, with appropriate assessment procedures, inpatient programmes and after care. In recognizing that such treatment is for a small minority, the rest of the book will describe the components of a community-based approach to drug misuse treatment.

## Summary

The threat which drug misuse poses to the well-being of society is partly due to its association with many related problems. 'Recreational' drug use is often defended on various grounds, notably that the currently legal substances may be more dangerous; but, as a behaviour, taking an illegal drug has a significantly antisocial element. In many cases usage is minor and transient, but persistent drug use is strongly associated with adolescent conduct problems, gang activities and various types of crime. While some drug misusers have predominantly psychological difficulties, in many the general effects of family disruption and a lack of social opportunities appear more important. Deprived areas in which there is aggregation of groups with various problems are fertile ground for drug suppliers, with young people in many such neighbourhoods encountering drugs routinely.

The drugs problem is addressed through various methods of prevention, education, treatment and enforcement. In treatment services we cannot possibly solve the wider social problems, and our first duty is to help, as effectively as we can, those who present to us wishing to reduce or stop taking drugs. We must also try to improve the situation of those affected by such use, including in the wider communities if possible. Specifically, treatments which reduce drug-related crime by individuals have the potential for improving life in neighbourhoods, but much associated crime is not simply to fund drug habits, and in major cities treatment would have to be on a huge scale to make an overall impression on drug scenes. We have to work 'outwards' from the individuals we treat, aiming to produce as many benefits as possible through policies which effectively reduce drug-related harm.

In maximizing the numbers of drug misusers who can receive treatment, the options of inpatient care and long-term residential rehabilitation are only indicated for a small minority. Nevertheless, some individuals who cannot manage to detoxify in the community can do so in a residential setting, and there may be other strong reasons for admission. There needs to be careful appraisal of the suitability of cases for elective inpatient detoxification, as many difficult individuals prove as problematic to manage as inpatients as in the community, and quick relapse after labour- and cost-intensive methods is particularly unfortunate. Mostly such problems are likely to occur where detoxification has been unrealistically attempted in a user who is more suitably a maintenance treatment candidate.

Part I

# Treatments

# Methadone maintenance: a medical treatment for social reasons?

## Introduction

Methadone occupies a position of huge prominence in drug misuse treatment. As a synthetic opioid drug, it not only provides direct and effective relief of opiate withdrawal symptoms, but it is accepted as a long-term treatment option in those with a significant history of opiate dependence. Its selection as the main treatment drug in these indications is largely based on three properties, as shown in Table 1.1.

The first two properties are fundamental to the use of methadone, ideally allowing a heroin user, for instance, to switch from injecting a drug in a rapid cycle of relieving withdrawal symptoms, to taking a medication by mouth which will keep him or her well all day. The noneuphoriant property is relative, and we will see in further discussions on response to methadone, rationales for alternative medications and safety of treatment, that this is the least straightforward of the benefits of methadone. Overall, however, the effect of methadone is to enable an opiate misuser to 'just feel normal', and in individuals who accept this, the treatment routinely produces excellent results, in reducing other drug use and in a wide range of health and social outcomes (Farrell et al. 1994, Bertschy 1995, Marsch 1998). The effectiveness of maintenance treatment makes up for the big relapse rates after detoxification from drugs, and is a major factor in the selective presentation of opiate users to drug services. The promotion of methadone maintenance at the time when HIV began spreading among drug misusers was testament to this effectiveness: methadone has nothing directly to do with HIV, but it engages drug misusers so that other harm reduction work can be done, and it is the simplest way of quickly reducing an individual's other drug use and injecting.

But what exactly are we doing when we prescribe methadone? Given the strong social basis of drug misuse, and the commonality of personal factors across misuse of the various drugs, it seems highly unlikely that there can be a definitive pharmacological treatment in the case of one, and only one, drug type. Is methadone a treatment, as such, which

Table 1.1. *Properties of methadone and resultant benefits in clinical treatment*

| Property | Benefit in treatment |
|---|---|
| Effective orally | Oral preparations, preferably liquid, enable cessation of injecting |
| Long acting | Avoids frequent withdrawal symptoms, may be taken once per day |
| Noneuphoriant | Stabilizing effect, relatively little temptation to over-use supply |

normalizes the behaviour and personal functioning of an addict, or is the media term 'heroin substitute' more appropriate? Is it simply that opiates are the most addictive drugs, *therefore* the method of substitution treatment is approved, *therefore* many indirect benefits occur as individuals are removed from the lifestyle of using illicit drugs? Whatever the mechanism by which methadone produces its results, further questions also arise. In so far as we are treating health problems, are they those of individuals or, since the approach aimed at HIV prevention, is the provision of methadone in effect a public health measure? Many of the most obvious benefits of methadone treatment in practice are firmly social, such as improved relationships, stopping crime or getting out of debt – how appropriate is a doctor's role in such circumstances?

This chapter considers different models of providing long-term methadone, and what they suggest about the nature of this treatment approach. There is a short review of studies of effectiveness, the most systematic of which mainly date from the early days of such treatment. The reasons which lie behind the gradual departure from the original model of methadone programmes are discussed, as are some of the limitations of the medication which have become apparent, particularly in its use in wider populations. The main practical issues which arise in current usage of methadone, and the prescribing of alternative forms, including injectable methadone, are also considered.

## The term 'methadone maintenance'

This term is used increasingly casually to refer to ongoing prescribing of methadone over any reasonably lengthy time period. Usually a constant dose is implied, but sometimes slowly reducing courses are also described in this way. Strictly speaking, however, the term refers to the highly structured programme approach which was originally devised for the delivery of methadone treatment in the USA, and is described next. This is not just a matter of semantics since, as we shall see, most of the systematic evidence for methadone's effectiveness relates to treatment as carried out in structured programmes, and the inference that any long-term prescribing amounts to approximately the same thing can lead to false assumptions about the process and its possible benefits.

## Formal methadone maintenance programmes

It is well known that the concept of formalized methadone maintenance originates from the work of Dole & Nyswander (1965). The treatment was devised for established opiate addicts, and was based on the principle that, following the physiological changes which occurred through prolonged taking of opiates, the state of dependence represented a metabolic disorder which required corrective treatment indefinitely. The fundamental aspect of methadone treatment was seen to be not simply the relief of withdrawal symptoms and craving, but a 'narcotic blockade', whereby an individual on methadone would fail to experience the euphoriant effects of heroin if that were taken (Dole et al. 1966). This effect was considered to be due to cross-tolerance, and it was observed that methadone doses of at least 80 mg per day were necessary to achieve it. This relatively high dose was therefore prescribed on a long-term basis, with no intention that patients should attempt to reduce. The first clinical programmes were for recidivist addicts, with the related aims of reducing heroin use and crime.

A structured programme approach to the delivery of methadone treatment was considered essential. Addicts were stabilized on high-dose methadone in a hospital ward, following which they returned on a daily basis for supervised consumption of medication and urine testing. There was an initial comprehensive assessment of medical, psychiatric and social problems, with facilities to address these on an ongoing basis. Along with the provision of methadone, the addicts entered not only counselling, but also placements in education or employment. Relaxation of the daily attendance for methadone or urine screening was only for individuals deemed to be making excellent progress, although take-home doses for part of the day were also necessary for those who had difficulty spanning a 24-hour period with one dose. Programmes along these lines developed across the USA, with inevitably some differences in provision emerging over the years. Ball & Ross (1991) undertook a clinical outcome study across six methadone programmes in the mid-1980s, and found a wide variation in programme elements and effectiveness. This research was considered to support strongly methadone treatment as it had been originally devised, with the most successful programmes characterized by high methadone doses, definite maintenance treatment rather than attempts at reduction, more intensive counselling and more medical services, as well as features indicating good relationships between staff and patients.

## Other long-term methadone prescribing

Since methadone was introduced it has, in practice, been provided according to a very wide range of treatment models and policies. There are major differences in treatment internationally, which are mainly beyond the scope of this book but have been the subject of reviews (Gossop & Grant 1991, Farrell et al. 1995). Notwithstanding the strong evidence for the original approach, which is discussed further below, there has generally been a gradual departure from this, for various reasons which are inter-related. The overall trends in provision have been towards lower dosage, fewer additional interventions and less acceptance of outright maintenance treatment although, importantly, these do not necessarily apply together.

The dilution of the original approach within the USA has been partly due to financial and political considerations (Rosenbaum 1995), but many other influences have also affected services. As with other psychiatric conditions, ideologically there has been less acceptance of the medical model, and therefore, in the case of methadone, of the implicit need for life-long treatment. In the meantime, heroin has become more and more available, with a wider range of individuals presenting, who may require a long-term approach but not necessarily a universal high-dose policy. Also, elements such as special employment schemes have become much less common and, without these, routine daily attendance at a treatment centre has gradually been considered less acceptable, for those who are attempting to normalize their lifestyle in other ways.

Some of the changes which have occurred in methadone treatment have come about as a result of the threat posed by the involvement of drug misusers in the HIV epidemic. In the UK and other countries methadone was seen as an important vehicle for shifting heroin users away from the risks of injecting (e.g. Advisory Council on the Misuse of Drugs 1988), but it was recognized that the delivery of treatment needed to be substantially altered if it was to make an impact in public health terms (see Chapter 7). There was much emphasis on engagement in treatment, with methadone in effect attracting users into services so that other HIV-preventive work could be undertaken, and also on subsequent retention, with routine discharge from treatment for additional drug use considered inappropriate. This use of methadone for individuals who would in many cases not previously have qualified for definite mainten-ance produced more instances of ongoing low-dose treatment, and the retention aspect meant that there was more recognition of those who do not successfully modify their drug use to taking methadone alone. Rigid approaches have been considered undesirable primarily because they may deter those individuals who pose some of the highest risks, while ideologi-cal considerations have been important in generally taking more account of individuals' views on their own treatment. In this way many 'low threshold' programmes have grown up (e.g. Buning et al. 1990, Klingemann 1996, Plomp et al. 1996) with the over-riding philosophies of easy access to treatment, harm reduction policies and individualized dosing.

Lower average doses of methadone have resulted not only from the drug being given to a broader population, but from heightened awareness of its side-effects and particular addictive potential. The addictiveness does not so much matter if treatment is conceived as being life-long, but relatively few patients in current treatment wish this to be the case. With abstinence often the ultimate aim, many individuals elect to be on the lowest comfortable dose of methadone with a view to gradual reduction, and something of a hybrid between maintenance and detoxification has emerged, variously referred to as short-term maintenance, 'maintenance to abstinence' (Department of Health 1991) or 'abstinence-orientated maintenance' (Capelhorn 1994). Outcomes in time-limited methadone treatment have generally been found to be very poor in comparison with maintenance (McGlothin & Anglin 1981, Rosenbaum et al. 1988), but studies have typically been in established maintenance candidates who have had treatment restricted, rather than individuals who have chosen to reduce as an option within a flexible policy. For our purposes this intermediate duration of treatment is classed as slow detoxification, and is discussed in the section on methadone detoxification in Chapter 3.

The elements of counselling and urine testing remain integral to long-term methadone provision in many services, although both to a lesser degree than in formal maintenance programmes. Both are dis-cussed below, but we should first consider a little further the nature of methadone treatment itself.

Table 1.2. *Medical model and substitution model of methadone treatment*

|  | Medical model | Substitution model |
|---|---|---|
| Rationale | To correct metabolic disturbance caused by opiate dependence | To provide a reasonably satisfying drug effect |
| Mechanism | Reduces craving and blocks effects of other opiates | Reduces need to use other drugs |
| Explanation for improvements in health and well being | Primary, due to methadone | Secondary, due to removal from street drug use |
| Dose | High | Minimum comfortable dose |
| Duration | Indefinite | Should be able to gradually withdraw |

## The nature of methadone treatment

### Specific treatment or heroin substitute?

A comparison between the medical model of methadone treatment and a model of methadone as a so-called heroin substitute is outlined in Table 1.2, and these concepts will now be considered.

The medical model of methadone treatment, as proposed by Dole & Nyswander (1965), has been reviewed more recently by their co-worker Kreek (1992). The initial studies pre-dated the discovery of the opiate receptors and endogenous opioids, and methadone was selected largely on the basis of careful clinical observation in pain patients and in addicts. The clinical properties of long duration of action (24–36 hours) and effectiveness by mouth were considered highly advantageous, and in addicts the drug appeared to reduce craving and produce a 'narcotic blockade', referred to above. This approach to opiate addiction was widely taken up in the USA and elsewhere, and in this original concept methadone is seen as a purely medical treatment, resembling the use of insulin in diabetes or antihypertensives in high blood pressure. The early proponents stressed that in cases where dependence had become clearly established over a significant period, the treatment should be continued for as long as the patient wished, and while it was producing benefit, with Dole (1973) asserting that 'each withdrawal [from methadone mainten-ance] is an experiment with the life of a patient'. It has frequently been pointed out that the portrayal of methadone as a straightforward medical approach has been particularly necessary in the USA politically, where the concept of a substitute drug would fit uneasily with the strong emphasis on enforcement. The suggestion in this version of treatment is that it is the medication itself which produces the behavioural changes, but the substitution process is still implicated, if methadone acts to reduce craving for other opiates and to deter such usage through its blockade effect.

Alternatively, the substitution principle may be spelt out rather more directly, as it tends to be in European countries. (In the UK we are often considered to have a specific 'British system', but this is largely a separate matter relating to drug legislation and prescribing before the modern era of recreational drug misuse, although the concept does include our use of some injectable medications (Strang & Gossop 1994).) Broadly, the 'heroin substitute' view of methadone regards the provision of a guaranteed supply of legal pharmaceutical opioid as leading to a range of secondary benefits, as the activity of illicit drug taking is reduced or stopped. Improvements in general health, mood and personality are therefore seen as indirect rather than direct effects of methadone, more related to avoiding the complications of other drug use. Indeed, methadone is truly a substitute for the preferred drug, heroin, and although the long-acting property and oral route are acknowledged as beneficial, in this view of methadone there is also more acceptance that individuals will actually vary greatly in their ability to adjust to methadone's much more limited subjective effects.

Although the concept of substitution is quite compatible with ongoing treatment, the issue of duration of methadone to some extent becomes tied in with treatment models. Thus, long-term maintenance is sometimes referred to as 'medical maintenance', and short-term treatment as 'psychotherapeutic maintenance'. The implication of the latter term is that with additional therapy and support it ought to be possible for an addict to be 'weaned off' opiates using a reducing course of methadone. This presupposes that opiate tolerance gradually reduces during withdrawal, in an opposite process to the increase which occurs as opiate dependence develops, whereas the medical model does not accept that the various neurobiological and neuroendocrine abnormalities in opiate dependence can in fact be reversed (Kreek 1992). This issue is far from clear-cut, as the medical model view is based substantially on the high relapse rates after detoxification, to which many kinds of factors may contribute, as well as on biological changes of uncertain clinical importance.

Such contrasting views of methadone treatment were encapsulated in a brief joint article in *Addiction* journal, which was followed by a series of commentaries (Ball & van de Wijngaart 1994, Wodak et al. 1994). On a visit during a harm reduction conference, Dr Ball, who has carried out some of the main work on beneficial elements of methadone mainten- ance programmes, and Dr Wijngaart, an expert on Dutch drug policy, had interviewed a client at the methadone clinic in Utrecht, The Nether- lands. In a frank discussion with the programme director and other visitors, the client described his many previous attempts to come off drugs, and related that he had reduced his methadone to 12.5 mg per day. He was not hopeful of completing his methadone reduction, but said that he was 38 years old and he wanted to be changing his life and seeing more of his two children. Unfortunately, as well as his methadone, he was still taking a wide range of other drugs by injection, and he believed that many other clients in the programme did the same. The two authors gave their different views of this situation, with Dr Ball regretting that 'some- what surprisingly, [the client] seems uninformed about the pharmacology of methadone maintenance and the need for long-term treatment'. Dr Wijngaart observed that the client was 'a typical Dutch methadone client', from a background of using many different kinds of drugs and probably quite unable to adhere to only methadone. Habitual drug users were entitled to 'seek detoxification to regain their health temporarily or because they really want to stop their drug dependence', but the main purpose of methadone was to keep a wide range of clients in contact so that other harm reduction measures could be deployed.

The issue of whether it is inadvisable to attempt to detoxify from methadone maintenance is a major and controversial one, but the study by Eklund et al. (1994) neatly illustrates some salient points. It was carried out in Sweden, within a USA-style methadone policy where there was no requirement to detoxify from established maintenance treatment. How- ever, 59 out of 600 patients had voluntarily done so, and their outcomes were investigated, at an average follow-up of seven years. The high number of seven had died, and two were untraceable. Of the remaining 50, 25 had successfully withdrawn from methadone, 19 at the first attempt. Of those, however, five had current substance misuse problems, mainly with alcohol. Twenty-five had resumed methadone maintenance and had usually achieved good stability, but quality of life measures were generally better in those who had succeeded in withdrawing from meth- adone. In this group who were very long-term drug users, therefore, it appeared that attempting to withdraw from maintenance treatment was risky, with a tendency to substitute with other substances, but that if it could be achieved, it resulted in a better quality of life.

In this book methadone is referred to as a substitution treatment, and that concept is generally employed rather than the purely medical model. It is considered that one of the main reasons why long-term methadone treatment produces such good results is that it does not require those who have risk factors for ongoing drug misuse, such as personality disorder or an adverse social situation, to be completely without the effects of a mood-altering drug, albeit that those effects are limited in the case of methadone. Further, it is relatively easy to avoid other substances of misuse, given that a drug is provided, and so there are consequent reductions in many other indices of drug use such as injecting or HIV-risk behaviours. Methadone is seen as being somewhat nonspecific in its impact on drug-taking patterns, but as a good starting point in attempts to convert individuals from street drug use to the clinically more desirable effects of a prescribed regime. It is clear that many opiate misusers cannot make this transition fully, and there need to be alternatives to simply discharging them from treatment, including other long-term prescribing options in some cases (see Chapter 2).

The nature of methadone treatment makes it unsurprising that retention rates are typically much higher than in other kinds of treatment for drug misuse. Methadone is a desirable commodity, and it must be acknowledged that this is not always for straightforward clinical reasons. Of course, well-motivated patients may routinely value all the various clinical benefits, but at the other end of the spectrum an individual may sell all their methadone to buy heroin, if given the chance. If this occurs the clinic is in effect giving currency, and there should be no surprise when such a patient reacts badly to this opportunity being curtailed if their 'medication' is reduced or stopped. Prevention of the abuse of services and medication ties in with the delivery of treatment, patient selection and the adequacy of monitoring, but the concept of methadone as a substitute drug helps explain the wide range of favourable responses on the part of patients towards this treatment approach. It is to be hoped that the extreme situation of a user diverting all their methadone is rare, but as security of treatment has generally been relaxed, we may hear of patients reserving their methadone for days on which they cannot get heroin, or selling a proportion of their prescription, the latter being most likely if there is a combination of high dosage but no supervision. The necessary security in treatment, and the difficulties in balancing this against making treatment accessible, are discussed in detail in Chapter 7.

The following case history illustrates several features which are reasonably characteristic of progress in treatment with methadone, as delivered in a community setting.

### Case history

Chris was a 24-year-old man who was single, but with a child from a previous relationship. He had an eight-year history of drug misuse, including cannabis, ecstasy, LSD and amphetamines, with heroin misuse for the past three years. He had initially smoked heroin, but progressed to injecting as he became more dependent, and at the time of referral was using 1–1.5 g per day. He had tried stopping several times himself, but had been unable to tolerate the withdrawal symptoms. He had had one methadone course from his general practitioner, but complained that this had reduced 'too quick', with heroin use restarting after the early stages.

It was agreed that Chris needed methadone treatment on a more prolonged basis. He was started on 60 mg per day, but an increase was required to 70 mg per day, on which he claimed to be entirely comfortable. He indicated that he did not want to be on methadone very long term, as he did not really see it as a solution, and believed it to be 'worse to get off than heroin'. There was no pressure from us to reduce quickly, and it was felt that an initial stabilizing period on the same dose was required.

At the first few appointments Chris' progress seemed excellent, with improvements in mood and general health. He was very pleased, and showed us the new clothes he had been able to buy with money which he said would have previously gone on drugs. While continuing at the same dose, however, his urine drug screens still showed heroin and, on one occasion, amphetamine, in addition to methadone. He told us his heroin use had dramatically declined, so that while he used to raise money illegally to buy heroin every day, he would now only have it if it was offered when somebody came round to his house. To his counsellor he admitted that although the methadone enabled him to avoid feeling ill, and he did not really crave heroin, there was something missing with the effect of methadone and he could not resist having different drugs on an occasional basis as a 'treat'. He retained a desire to change his lifestyle so that he was not involved in the drug scene, and he was sceptical of the idea that an increase in methadone would help him stop his other drug use.

It was agreed that Chris' situation had greatly improved on methadone treatment, but he was advised that for his methadone to continue, we would need to see his urine become free of nonprescribed drugs. Chris felt that such a requirement would actually help him in his own efforts to avoid other usage. Three out of four urine samples since have shown only methadone, and while one showed heroin, he emphasized that this was an isolated occasion and that he managed to smoke the drug rather than inject it. Overall, the reduction in Chris' drug use and criminal behaviour has been evident enough for his ex-girlfriend to allow him to have contact again with his young son. So far he has wished to remain on the same dose of methadone, and given the gains and the previous difficulties, this is considered appropriate at present.

## Individual treatment or public health policy?

The issue in considering this dimension is not so much whether benefits to individual health or public health accrue with methadone treatment, as clearly both do, and both are important in different ways. Partly the difficulty is whether, if we have one eye on the public health agenda of reducing HIV transmission from drug misusers, we can still apply the treatment that is best at any time for each individual. Since awareness of the risks of this particular infectious complication has been heightened, opiate misusers have in effect been 'cushioned' by the use of methadone treatment. They are already unlike all other types of drug misuser in being prescribed a closely related drug and, depending on treatment policies, in not being required to work towards abstinence; now methadone is also relied upon for engagement purposes, and to protect against relapses which might increase risk behaviours.

In relation to individuals and treatment populations, methadone has been shown not only to reduce other drug use and injecting, but specifically to reduce HIV risk behaviours (Darke et al. 1990, Capelhorn & Ross 1995, Marsch 1998), and sero-conversion rates (Metzer et al. 1993). Because of these impressive aspects, access to methadone treatment is generally encouraged, and in a low-threshold programme relatively few demands may be made. Criteria for receiving methadone are often not rigorous and, once in treatment, if it broadly appears that the harm-reduction aims are being met, there is a tendency for prescribing to 'drift' into the long term in individuals who are not definite maintenance candidates. This situation is compounded by the fact that public health-orientated treatment means maximum number of methadone patients, shorter appointments, less attention to individual drug-using situations, and less associated counselling to consider alternative management possibilities.

Even in undoubted long-term treatment, there is an uneasy mix between individualized treatment and the wider health and social aspects, as Raistrick (1997) points out in a thoughtful article on the subject. Although he acknowledges that 'prescribing methadone as a public health or social policy measure is not necessarily incompatible with prescribing for individual treatment', he envisages a situation where different purchasers of health care might have different desired outcomes, which would in turn influence the nature of substitution treatment. A criminal justice system purchaser might fund some places with the express aim of reducing the harm caused by criminal activity, and so to maximize that outcome prescribing would probably be high dose, long duration and include the possibility of injectable drugs or diamorphine if they were more effective for individuals in that regard. Furthermore, if an individual was failing on treatment there would be a tendency to go 'up the tariff' or, at the very least, retain them in the programme. By contrast, a patient on an individual treatment 'ticket' could face discharge from the programme for similar lack of progress, if the goal was more to encourage progressive reduction of dependency. At present 'in the real world prescribing doctors are pragmatists, and the circle is squared behind the closed door of the consulting room' (Raistrick 1997), but increasingly 'a transparency of objectives' is required in our understanding of the various purposes of methadone treatment. The irony is pointed out that methadone is usually paid for solely by health services, whereas the benefits extend widely into other areas, and it is rightly suggested that the criminal justice system and social services should also shoulder the financial burden, even if differential objectives would mean some adjustments in treatment methods.

Of the various possible roles of methadone treatment, the public health role which has been so strongly emphasized in the era of the HIV threat is requiring reassessment in the light of high prevalence rates of hepatitis C among injecting drug users (Wodak 1997, Serfaty et al. 1997). Although there have been many demonstrations of benefits of methadone maintenance in relation to indicators of HIV risk, the hepatitis C rates suggest transmission of this agent has still occurred and this is much more transmissible than HIV through blood (although less so through sexual contact). Different kinds of injecting equipment sharing are implicated, and it seems that some of the behaviour changes advised to reduce HIV risk are not sufficient to avoid hepatitis C (Wells 1998). In a study giving cause for concern, Crofts et al. (1997) found that methadone maintenance treatment failed to protect against new acquisition of hepatitis C in a significant proportion of cases, and further similar investigations will be required to judge the impact of methadone on this additional serious health problem.

## Effectiveness of methadone

Comprehensive reviews of the effectiveness of methadone have been provided by several authors (Hall et al. 1998, Farrell et al. 1994, Bertschy 1995, Marsch 1998). Here, we will examine the subject enough to gauge the overall importance of methadone for services, and to make some links with the discussions of the nature of the treatment and its practical provision.

It is extremely problematic adequately to undertake randomized controlled trials of substitution treatments in this specialty. Drug misusers are not going to have neutral views as to whether they receive methadone or no treatment or, say, methadone or intravenous diamorphine. Apart from the issues of consent, methadone is now of a status such that it would usually be considered unethical to withhold it from users who had a clinical need. Because of the difficulties, the evidence which so strongly supports methadone maintenance is largely from observational studies which back up a small number of early randomized trials.

The reviews mentioned above make it clear that the majority of studies demonstrating the effectiveness of methadone are of ongoing maintenance treatment. The evidence generally becomes weaker as duration of treatment shortens, through to detoxification treatments. In services we may choose to do short-term treatment and, importantly, users themselves will often choose it, but it cannot be considered to be supported by much systematic evidence. Furthermore, the evidence also weakens as there is departure from the original model of formal methadone maintenance programmes, no doubt confirming the worst suspicions of those who feel that current models of providing methadone are misguided. In defence of the various relatively unstructured treatment methods, it should be pointed out that the major studies were carried out many years ago in highly selected populations, and may be of limited relevance in terms of current heroin usage and the revised purposes of methadone treatment. Although the importance of additional programme elements is often stressed (Ball & Ross 1991), the provision of the drug itself has been seen as the single most important aspect ever since the first trials of structured methadone treatment (Dole & Nyswander 1965), and the outcomes in studies most strongly relate to direct drug factors, such as duration or dosage. Studies of methadone detoxification, mainly in the UK context, are discussed in Chapter 3, but the following are some important studies of maintenance treatment.

Randomized controlled trials have necessarily been carried out in rather atypical situations where methadone treatment was not otherwise available, so that those randomized to no treatment would not receive the drug elsewhere. The first was by Dole et al. (1969) in recidivist opiate addicts who were due for release from prison. Entry criteria included at least a four-year history of opiate addiction and at least one previous unsuccessful rehabilitation attempt. Twelve individuals started methadone treatment, with 16 randomized to no treatment, and at 12 months the findings were overwhelmingly in favour of methadone maintenance. Indeed, all of the control sample had returned to daily heroin use and prison, while none of the methadone patients was using heroin daily and only three had been imprisoned. A larger study in a broader population was carried out in Hong Kong, where methadone treatment was not otherwise available (Newman & Whitehill 1979). The same entry criteria were used, with evidence of daily opiate use, and 100 male addicts were included. All subjects were stabilized in hospital on 60 mg of methadone per day, and were randomly assigned either to be withdrawn from methadone under double-blind conditions and then receive placebo maintenance, or to receive methadone maintenance, both groups also having additional counselling treatments. Methadone maintenance dose was determined by the patients and averaged 97 mg per day, and those who had more than six urine tests positive for heroin during the follow-up, or who missed six daily doses, were discharged from the programme. At 32 weeks only 5 of the 50 placebo subjects were still in treatment, as against 38 of the 50 methadone subjects, the pattern continuing to produce figures of 1 and 28 respectively at three years. A significantly greater proportion of the placebo group than the methadone group had been discharged for heroin use, but three deaths had all been in the methadone group.

A study in Sweden used similar entry criteria (Gunne & Gronbladh 1981), but added a period of intensive inpatient vocational rehabilitation to the methadone maintenance programme, and employed a sequential design. Once again, at follow-up after two years almost none of the control group had ceased drug use or made other satisfactory progress, while in the treatment group there were high levels of cessation of other drugs and gaining employment or further education. A further randomized controlled study by Yancovitz et al. (1991) is interesting in that it tested the effects of 'interim' methadone treatment, involving limited other services, in those awaiting treatment in comprehensive methadone programmes. Treatment subjects received high-dose oral methadone by daily dispensing, but no counselling or structured social rehabilitation. A total of 301 heroin addicts were recruited, and in the period of interim treatment the proportion of subjects receiving methadone who were shown by urinalysis to be using heroin declined from 63% to 29%, with no corresponding decrease in the control sample. There was, however, no change in cocaine use in either group.

The Treatment Outcome Prospective Study (Hubbard et al. 1984, Hubbard et al. 1989) included over 11 000 drug misusers who had applied for treatment programmes in the USA over a three-year period. The treatment approaches were grouped into methadone maintenance, residential therapeutic communities, and outpatient drug-free counselling, and there was an extensive series of follow-up interviews, some on selected subgroups of clients. The outcome measures in the study were illicit drug use, criminal activity, employment, depression and suicide, and statistical techniques were used to control for various confounding factors such as educational level and extent of previous treatment. This study forms some of the basis for the often-quoted view that results of treatment are generally better the longer that individuals stay in the treatment, as that applied to various outcomes in this research. Retention rates were significantly better in methadone maintenance than the other modalities, and regular heroin use and crime in that group both dropped from high levels to less than 10% of individuals, 1–3 months into treatment.

Higher methadone dosages have been found in various studies to be associated with less heroin use and improved retention in treatment (e.g. Ling et al. 1976, Ball & Ross 1991, Joe et al. 1991). In an Australian maintenance programme, Capelhorn and colleagues have demonstrated a greatly increased risk of leaving treatment among those prescribed less than 60 mg per day compared with those prescribed up to 80 mg per day (Capelhorn & Bell 1991), and an inverse relationship between additional heroin use and methadone dose, between 40 mg and 80 mg per day (Capelhorn et al. 1993). However, the contradictory results of Seow et al. (1980) suggest that benefits of high dosage are not necessarily demonstrable where that is reserved for individuals who have failed on low dosage, since they may to some extent represent a more difficult group who are prone anyway to additional drug use. Hartel et al. (1995) found that heroin use was generally greater in those who were maintained on less than 70 mg of methadone per day, but that patients who used cocaine were more likely than others to use heroin at all methadone dosage levels.

In the reviews cited at the start of this section there is some breakdown of findings into those relating to heroin use, criminality, HIV-risk behaviours, social rehabilitation and nonopiate abuse. We have noted that crime was one of the earliest indicators in methadone treatment, while the wider range of outcomes is formalized in current drug misuse rating instruments such as the Opiate Treatment Index (Darke et al. 1992a). The main areas in which methadone treatment has been found to be of substantial benefit are indicated in Table 1.3.

The list gives the approximate order in which effects have been demonstrated in systematic studies, according to reviews of studies and a recent meta-analysis (Marsch 1998). There is clearly a very substantial social component to beneficial treatment outcomes, with quality of life, for instance, including family and personal relationships, social stability, finances and other aspects of social functioning. These are commonly among the main areas of improvement seen in clinical practice, behind the most direct effects of reduced opiate misuse and drug-related crime. The demonstration in studies of methadone patients gaining employment has generally decreased over time, probably due to fewer special schemes and the wider unemployment picture, with some differences found between countries. Reduction in use of nonopiate drugs by individuals on methadone is undoubtedly very variable, with studies in general suggesting overall benefit, but in practice some problematic combinations with alcohol, benzodiazepines, cocaine and other drugs which are discussed elsewhere in this book. The data on mortality partly relies on comparisons with out-of-treatment drug misusers, including those refused treatment or discharged, who may differ in important ways from those who are retained; this subject is discussed in detail in Chapter 7. More limited is the evidence of an impact of methadone on HIV-risk sexual behaviours, as opposed to injecting practices (Stark et al. 1996). This discrepancy, found in many studies, is unsurprising, but needs to be acknowledged in view of the emphasis on methadone as an HIV-preventative measure. Also, there are many subgroups of drug misusers who are relatively unlikely to adopt even the safe injecting practices, such as those with antisocial personality disorder, other psychiatric problems, benzodiazepine abuse or various characteristic patterns of drug using with peers (Darke 1998).

In Table 1.3 I have included the areas of physical and psychological health, which often do not feature in reviews. Methadone has significant adverse effects, as discussed below, and by no means do all patients report subjective improvements in health on the drug, as opposed to when taking street heroin or other opiates. However, if methadone treatment is

Table 1.3. *Main areas of benefit in methadone treatment*

| |
| --- |
| Reduced opiate misuse |
| Reduced crime and imprisonment |
| Reduced HIV risk behaviours (injecting) |
| Improved quality of life |
| Improved physical and psychological health |
| Reduced nonopiate misuse |
| Employment, college |
| Reduced death rate |
| Reduced HIV risk behaviours (sexual) |

adhered to, there is normalization of various circadian rhythms and endocrine effects including menstruation (Kreek 1992, American Psychiatric Association 1994), and improved immunological function, possibly relevant in delaying progression of HIV disease (McLachlan et al. 1993). In addition, the various complications of injecting and of erratically using street drugs can be avoided. Improvements in psychological functioning, such as reduced anxiety, depression and other mood disturbances, have also been reported (Musselman & Kell 1995).

Before leaving the subject of the general effectiveness of methadone, two further general points should be made regarding the evidence from studies. One is that the cohorts of methadone patients in strict programmes are self-selecting, with discharge from the programme if there is persistent use of other drugs. Some studies make adjustment for this, but in many, the improvements seen are in the subgroups who were able to adhere to the desired position of taking methadone only. Also, the influential early studies often excluded those with a significant history of polydrug use (Dole et al. 1969, Gunne & Gronbladh 1981). In many areas polydrug use is the norm in those presenting for treatment, including those accepted for methadone, because of the extent of predominant opiate use (Bell et al. 1990a). Such individuals are likely to differ substantially from those in the original studies in terms of treatment needs and response to standardized methadone treatment.

## Associated counselling

Counselling is one of the main aspects of process which has been examined in studies of methadone treatment. In general, once again, the most positive evidence is in favour of a systematic and comprehensive approach. McLellan et al. (1993) randomly assigned 92 methadone patients to three groups which differed in levels of psychosocial services, with the actual methadone treatment remaining the same. Some 69% of subjects who received virtually only the methadone prescription continued to use other opiates or cocaine, with lower levels in groups who received additional counselling (41%), or counselling plus on-site medical and psychiatric services, workshops on employment skills and family therapy (19%). There is also some evidence supporting the addition to methadone maintenance of motivational interviewing (Saunders et al. 1995), and a therapeutic community-orientated day programme (De Leon et al. 1997). The low acceptability of formal psychotherapy in drug misusers has been recognized (Seivewright & Daly 1997), and was strikingly illustrated in a controlled trial of short-term interpersonal psychotherapy by Rounsaville et al. (1983). Only 5% of eligible patients agreed to participate in that trial, with around half of subjects completing the study treatment. Better results were shown in a study where the therapy was cognitive–behavioural in nature rather than dynamic (McLellan et al. 1986).

A study which appears important in demonstrating that intensive treatment is not necessary for all methadone patients is that by Senay et al. (1993). In a controlled comparison, some individuals who had progressed very well in methadone treatment were switched from a conventional intensive regime to a system of having medical and counselling appointments only monthly, with other relaxations in programme elements. Not only was stability maintained, as demonstrated by a range of outcome measures and urine testing, but the new approach was so much preferred that it was considered unethical to return those users to the more demanding regime. The authors observed that, for well stabilized patients, 'the time spent in travelling to a clinic two or three times a week and then waiting in lines for methadone and / or for counselling . . . creates problems in getting or holding a job and significantly limits their ability to relate to their family. In addition, they are exposed constantly to non-recovering patients and experience this as additionally burdensome, as these are the very people they are trying to avoid.'

Following the evolution of methadone treatment internationally, as summarized earlier in the chapter, in many clinics medical and counselling appointments are at about that monthly frequency, with counselling mainly on an individual basis. In our experience it is preferable to have the two kinds of appointments as separate, with the counsellor spending some of his or her time discussing the methadone treatment, but also looking at wider personal and lifestyle aspects. The actual combination of appointments depends on staffing and other considerations, and often it is not possible for all patients to have a counsellor as well as a prescriber. Having only a prescriber risks neglect of aspects such as lifestyle planning, family support or consideration of other treatments; but, at the same time, if resources are limited, counselling needs to be targeted for those who will derive most benefit. The worst scenario, which needs to be guarded against, is where a methadone patient fails to attend for organized counselling, and uses the counsellor only as a contact at other times over specific and possibly manipulative prescription-related requests.

## Practical management

In common with many other clinics in the UK, in our own services we tread something of a middle path between the formalized programmes and the low-threshold, low-demand approach to methadone treatment. There is no establishment of a structured programme with the various additional on-site services and, even if that were advocated, the funding climate generally is such that it could not realistically be provided. Ours are community-orientated services, with treatment mainly delivered through our specialist multidisciplinary clinical team and associated staff. The services are described further in Chapter 5.

Approximately 25% of our patients are on long-term methadone, with criteria for its use based on broad general guidance (Department of Health 1991, American Psychiatric Association 1994): established physical dependence on opiates (usually heroin), at least two years of opiate use, previous unsuccessful experience of detoxification treatment (or clearly severe history if no such prior treatment), and preferably aged 18 years or over, although exceptions are necessary to this. Usually methadone mixture is used, in dosages of 40–120 mg per day, with dispensing at community pharmacies. We emphasize that methadone should replace heroin use rather than be additional to it, and encouragement, counselling and monitoring are provided with that aim. To some extent the requirements on patients depend on the nature and extent of their prescribed medication, which principle is discussed at various stages in this book, and outright discharge from treatment for additional drug use is relatively rare.

In such treatment there are various important practical considerations, and some of the main principles are examined here. More detail is provided on practical aspects in the discussion of the use of methadone as a detoxification treatment in Chapter 3.

**Treatment contracts**
The nature of methadone treatment makes some kind of contract between patient and clinic essential. These may be in standard form for everybody, or individualized according to the particular circumstances of cases. Many services prefer contracts to be in writing and signed, although an unambiguous verbal agreement with recording in the case notes is basically as satisfactory. The most fundamental aspect is the required abstinence from other drugs of misuse which, as we have noted, varies to some extent in different approaches to methadone treatment. In practice we find it suitable to operate something of a hierarchy in contractual obligations depending on the prescribed medication: an individual on high-dose methadone or injectable drugs is required to be completely abstinent from other drugs, and has a generally stricter contract in matters such as frequency of dispensing, whereas there may not be quite the same expectations in someone who has elected to be on low-dose oral methadone.

The other elements which need to be included in contracts, and approaches to contract breaches, are outlined on page 94, and mainly apply to both maintenance and detoxification treatment. Although it can seem paradoxical, sanctions should include reductions in methadone dose where this appears the only way of making an impact on additional drug-taking or other problematic behaviours. In our long-term treatment we consider it inadvisable to specify exact lengths of time an individual is to be on a certain prescription, as changes may be required for various reasons, but it should be made clear that treatment will continue provided the contract is adhered to.

**Urine testing**
It can correctly be said that the evidence from studies regarding benefit of urine testing over patient self-reporting of drug use is not very convincing (Ward et al. 1998a). However, it must be noted that the comparisons were mainly carried out in the early maintenance programmes where patients were observed every day when presenting for their methadone, a far cry from a modern clinic where there may only be contact monthly. In our view urine testing is essential at every appointment, simply because it usually provides the only objective evidence of progress. In the early days 'random' urine testing meant that the patient still provided a sample

every day but only some from each week were tested, whereas currently if samples are only taken at some appointments, long periods can go by without any information. Giving a urine sample is not a demanding requirement in exchange for treatment of this nature, and it should not be made possible for users to avoid it. We find no problem with acceptance of this policy, providing the same applies to everybody.

The main limitation of urine testing is that most of the street drugs stay detectable for only 2–4 days after testing. It is important to have the local laboratory's guidance on their own assays available, so that there can be confidence when discussing the results with patients. Typically, benzodiazepines remain detectable for longer, although they are difficult to identify individually, and cannabis poses particular problems due to patchy excretion over a long period. (It is perhaps fortunate that cannabis is relatively rarely made the subject of a treatment contract, at least in outpatients.) The short period of detection of the main drugs of misuse leads to scepticism that, even within a strict treatment contract, users may simply 'clean up their act' for four days before their appointment, but demonstrable clean urines are still a good starting point, and the habit of such abstinence may then extend to longer periods. Steps must be taken to reduce the chances of giving false samples, such as checking temperature and colour, and avoiding having several patients giving samples at the same time, but many clinics, including ours, usually stop short of direct observation.

Systems for 'instant' urine testing clearly offer the general advantage that information can be available without delay, at times when treatment is to be initiated or changes may be necessary. Reluctance to employ such systems fully appears to have been due to considerations such as the additional role for the drug worker – especially where time-consuming multiple assays are required for different drugs – and the problem of using results of slightly questionable reliability in situations such as imposing treatment sanctions, as well as to the matter of expense. Techniques and reliability are continually improving, with immunoassay detection of multiple drugs from one sample now available, and there are many clinical situations in which instant testing is highly desirable, such as checking opiate-free status before starting naltrexone. In ongoing methadone treatment (and other instances), the presence of instant testing probably reduces the likelihood of misrepresentation by patients at appointments, and if clinicians are satisfied with the reliability the whole process of monitoring adherence to treatment contracts is made more direct. Laboratory testing means that clinicians are always working with a lag in available results, but if this is the only method used a way must be devised of adjusting to it. In ongoing methadone treatment, therefore, rather than authorizing prescriptions for the whole period until the next appointment, the initial period until receipt of the result can be covered, with the remaining prescriptions conditional on the result. Hair testing for drugs, with a sample easily obtained, confers several advantages over urine (McPhillips et al. 1998), most notably in the period over which drugs are detectable, which is basically as long as the hair grows. It is not used routinely in clinical practice but, increasingly, drugs services and other agencies such as social services involved in child care cases, and probation, are becoming aware that this method is indicated where it is essential to know whether individuals are using drugs on an ongoing basis.

**Additional medication**
As far as possible, methadone treatment should mean just that, not methadone plus other medications of potential misuse. The theoretical footing for this is that the majority of the positive evidence for effectiveness relates to methadone alone, although we noted earlier that the main studies did not include individuals who were significant users of nonopiate drugs.

Those of us in countries where high-dose methadone maintenance is not unequivocally promoted must concede that we are likely to have more difficulties with additional psychoactive medication use in treatment. The most problematic drugs are the benzodiazepines, which are taken partly to enhance the effect of methadone (Stitzer et al. 1981, Preston et al. 1984, Griffiths & Weerts 1997), that combination therefore being more 'necessary' at lower dose. In our clinics we generally aim to eliminate benzodiazepine misuse, but in those who wish to avoid a high methadone dosage and are capable of stabilizing, or who fail to respond to psychological treatment of associated anxiety problems, prescribing of benzodiazepines is sometimes accommodated. Unfortunately there are some individuals who will still use benzodiazepines even on high-dose methadone, and these difficult clinical situations are discussed further in the section on prescribing benzodiazepines in Chapter 2. Given the nature of drug misuse clinics, any prescribing of benzodiazepines to some individuals will result in others seeking to obtain them without clinical need, and so, as with the opioid drugs, a clinic-wide policy is as important to establish as the individualized treatment regimes.

Indications for other psychotropic medication such as antidepressants and antipsychotics are basically the same as in other patients, but practical aspects are important. The drugs may not be able to be included in the same prescribing and dispensing arrangements as methadone, but a drug misuse clinic which is psychiatrically-based will often wish to take these on from the primary care physician, to more easily ensure regular control. The risks of inappropriate usage also apply to items such as analgesics or nutrition supplements, but there may need to be some sharing of prescribing for financial or other reasons. In cases of dual diagnosis with severe mental illness it is preferable for a general psychiatry service to be involved with aspects such as depot antipsychotic medication, but this may fall to the drug misuse service if there is better compliance at the methadone clinic.

### Behaviour problems

Several factors combine to make behavioural disturbance at drug misuse clinics relatively likely. Attenders may be in states of some desperation, and they know that the clinic has the means to help them. At any presentation users may be either withdrawing or intoxicated, while as a group drug misusers have high levels of antisocial and aggressive behaviours, and low frustration tolerance. Staff must act in a professional manner which sets a good example, with appropriate assertiveness as necessary. The clinic should be available only for patients and those who essentially need to attend with them, and other associates may have to be turned away. Any instructions for attenders should be clear and unambiguous, with no misinformation.

The treatment contract should make it clear that aggression or abusiveness will not be tolerated in a clinic or home visit situation, and this requirement must be adhered to. Drug workers and clinic staff are also well placed to undertake general behavioural 'shaping', by failing to reinforce not only bogus requests for medication, but also various characteristic ploys such as disputing appointment times, involving others for manipulative purposes, seeking to gain advantage by disruptive behaviour, or even false financial claims. Residential rehabilitation centres see tackling such 'addict behaviours' as part of therapy, and other workers can certainly incorporate some elements of this approach.

Potential flashpoints for aggressive or disruptive behaviour should be recognized. Clearly, some patients are more likely to show this than others, but the situations are also predictable to some extent. Users are literally dependent on the clinic, and any failures in our arrangements can be badly received. Continuity in methadone treatment must be virtually guaranteed in normal circumstances, but beyond that it is perceived injustices regarding medication which provoke the most reaction. These can include being denied replacements of medication, discontent with a prescribing decision, or having a medication stopped on the grounds of breach of contract. Contracts must be very clear in this regard, especially concerning the circumstances in which a prescription initiated by the clinic would be retracted.

### Adverse effects

The most serious direct risks of methadone treatment are from overdosage, which are considered in detail in Chapter 7 and are heightened by combined use with other drugs. Otherwise, methadone appears to be remarkably safe for long-term use, causing no recognizable functional deficits or somatic damage (Kreek 1978). Novick et al. (1993) compared the health status of 110 patients who had been in methadone maintenance treatment for at least ten years with a control group of long-term heroin addicts, and found no clustering of unusual medical complications or abnormal laboratory results in the methadone group. Patients often need reassuring on this point, as many have the idea that methadone causes damage to liver, kidneys or other systems.

There are a range of more 'minor' adverse effects, however, which are often not mentioned in formal reviews of methadone treatment but which are discussed more in practical handbooks (e.g. Preston 1996a). In clinical practice these can be extremely problematic, variously leading to distress for individuals, limitations in compliance, and requests for alternative treatments, and the most troublesome such effects are listed in Table 1.4.

The full list of adverse effects of methadone resembles those of morphine, as they are common to the opiate group. These include nausea, vomiting, dizziness, mental clouding, dysphoria, euphoria, constipation, increased biliary tract pressure, respiratory depression, drying of respiratory secretions, sweating, lymphocytosis, and increased plasma concentrations of prolactin, albumin and globulins. Tolerance may develop more slowly to methadone than to morphine with respect to the depressant and sedative effects, which is linked to some of the dangers in the early stages of treatment (see Chapter 7) and problems of sedation clinically. Effects that are possibly more associated with methadone than other opiates include lethargy, feelings of heaviness in arms and legs, itching and other skin problems.

In the course of clinical treatment with methadone, certain situations

Table 1.4. *Main adverse effects of*
*methadone*

| |
| --- |
| Constipation |
| Sweating |
| Weight gain |
| Dental problems |
| Nausea |
| Amenorrhoea |
| Depression/lethargy |
| Reduced sexual desire |

relating to adverse effects are characteristic. Nausea is a general opiate effect, but complaints most frequently relate to the methadone mixture. This preparation does have a syrupy constituency, but the problem for clinicians is that the alternatives – sugar-free mixture or methadone tablets – are both more injectable, and therefore requests or implied requirements for these are often manipulative. So are requests for the antiemetic cyclizine tablets, which are crushed and injected by drug misusers and should not be given to this population, particularly as the usual form of abuse is in combination with injected methadone (see Chapter 4).

The other adverse effects which are commonly complained of in relation to methadone mixture in particular are weight gain and dental problems. Weight gain can be striking, as illustrated below but, contrary to frequent suggestions, cannot be accounted for by the calorie content of the mixture, as a 50 mg dose is apparently equivalent in this way to eating about two biscuits. There is therefore no indication to switch to an alternative form of methadone on these grounds, and it appears that the reasonably strong association between obesity and methadone treatment (Novick et al. 1993) may be due to a direct effect of the drug. Other relevant factors are that heroin addicts in treatment generally gain weight as they stop injecting and encountering chronic infections and develop a more sedentary lifestyle, although arguably in the case of methadone the latter may be associated with the lethargy that many patients complain of. In practice, we find that very excessive weight gain virtually only occurs in patients who are on high-dose methadone (over about 80 mg per day) and are mainly avoiding street drugs. In lesser degrees, weight gain is a reasonable general indicator of compliance with treatment, although some individuals do not experience it, presumably due to constitutional factors.

Regarding dental decay, methadone mixture is a culprit, because of the reduction in saliva, an effect of the acid on tooth enamel, and syrup constituents leading to the growth of plaque (Bigwood & Coehelho 1990). Once again, however, the situation is not straightforward, as there may be high consumption of snack foods, poor oral hygiene, infrequent attendance for dental check-ups or treatment, and masking of tooth ache by opiates. If alternatives to methadone mixture are considered unsuitable, patients can be advised to drink methadone through a straw or clean their teeth after taking it.

The side effects listed in Table 1.4 are generally those which cause most distress to individuals in treatment. Unfortunately, there are few useful treatments, so that in constipation the best approach is a high fibre diet and high (nonalcoholic) fluid intake. Sweating seems only partly accounted for by the histamine release, with other mechanisms produced by methadone likely. Amenorrhoea is due to high circulating prolactin levels and has the effect that pregnancy is often only recognized relatively late. Some couples falsely believe that pregnancy is not possible on opiates or methadone, and need advising on this point. There may be reduced sexual desire, which ties in with complaints of lethargy and depressed mood, although sexual dysfunctions may also be present (Spring et al. 1992).

In their generally favourable study, Novick et al. (1993) found an increased rate of diabetes mellitus in methadone maintenance patients, which they ascribed to the same causes as the obesity finding, namely high calorie intake and sedentary lifestyle.

### Case history

Stefan is a 26-year-old patient in our methadone clinic. He had been dependent on heroin for five years before presenting to the service, and clearly required substitution treatment on a probable long-term basis. His heroin usage was substantial and although, in the early stages of treatment, we attempted to manage him on 80 mg of methadone mixture per day, he required increases to 120 mg per day in the ensuing months. He felt that this dose was satisfactory, in that he was free of any withdrawal symptoms and felt mentally well, with no strong desire to use heroin. Occasionally, urine samples would show that he had used the drug, but this proved to be mainly on the days he received his benefit money, and he responded well to being advised that we would not tolerate such use on top of his methadone prescription. For the past year his only additional drug use has been of benzodiazepines, on an irregular basis.

Stefan has always had a big build, previously being an active sportsman.

However, whereas his usual weight had been around 210 lb, this has increased on methadone to 330 lb. This is the source of distress to him and more particularly to his wife, who finds his appearance embarrassing, especially as he has also developed excessive sweating. When questioned, Stefan states that he has little energy and rarely undertakes any physical activity, although this is compounded by the fact that he is reluctant to leave the house. He claims not to eat excessively in general, but he has a craving for sweet foods and has some chocolate every day.

Despite the problems, Stefan cannot contemplate being without methadone, or even reducing his dosage, which he unsuccessfully attempted at one stage. He feels that his life has improved in all other ways since giving up heroin, and he is fearful of risking a return to the drug-misusing lifestyle. He accepts the physical side effects, and in reality has little motivation to attempt weight reduction, for instance at a gym or a class. In view of his general satisfaction and his strong dependence on methadone, alternative approaches are not considered realistic at present.

## Other forms of methadone, including injectable

### Liquids

The form of methadone usually used in addiction practice is the mixture, 1 mg in 1 ml. In the UK addicts often mistakenly refer to this as linctus, but the linctus is a different strength preparation, 2 mg in 5 ml. The linctus can be useful when individuals are at very low methadone dose, since measurement is easier, but alternatively the mixture can be diluted. As noted above, a sugar-free version of the mixture can be used in those concerned about dental problems, calorie intake or nausea, although the grounds are not strong, and the sugar-free form is easier to abuse by injection. More concentrated liquids (e.g. 10 mg in 1 ml) are particularly useful for automatic dispensing machines.

### Tablets

The 5 mg tablets tend to prove unduly popular with patients if they are made available. Sometimes the reasons are genuine, such as carrying tablets to work rather than a bottle of liquid, but the tablets are also both more sellable and more injectable. They are a better proposition to sell as they can be seen to be unadulterated (whereas mixture may have been diluted), and so with the risk of their being crushed and injected, and with no real benefit of tablets for services, their prescribing in the UK is increasingly discouraged. As regards complaints of inability to take the mixture because of nausea, a policy of offering methadone suppositories in those circumstances dramatically reduces such claims!

Steels et al. (1992) reported their experience of attempting a change in prescribing policy, from the use of methadone tablets to methadone mixture, in a large UK clinic. The change aroused extreme hostility, with a rise in threatening behaviour towards staff. Wider effects included increases in the number of pharmacy burglaries and in the street value of methadone tablets, and the change was ultimately unsuccessful, with over three-quarters of the patients receiving tablets again three months later. Vomiting was the most common claimed adverse effect of mixture, but this was confirmed in only two cases.

**Injectable ampoules**
In the general discussions of methadone, we have noted that one of the most advantageous clinical properties is that it can be taken orally. There are a proportion of patients, however, who manifestly cannot give up injecting, and in such cases the use of methadone ampoules may be considered at least preferable to injecting street drugs. The treatment therefore perpetuates the aspect of injecting, and so the clinician must be certain that advantages accrue from the treatment which outweigh this. The usual circumstance would be that evidence of complete absence of street drug use is required for injectable methadone to be continued. Almost inevitably, before this treatment is used, there will have been prolonged failure to progress on oral methadone, with harmful injected use of other drugs which has a prospect of being eliminated if the step-up is made to injectable treatment.

In a survey of community pharmacies in the UK, Strang et al. (1996) found that of 3593 methadone prescriptions 80% were for oral liquid, 11% for tablets and 9% for injectable ampoules. The prescribing of ampoules has emerged as a pragmatic approach for intractable injectors, and there have been no controlled clinical trials. Policy-makers envisage that pa- tients may be started on injectable methadone and then encouraged to convert to the oral form (e.g. Advisory Council on the Misuse of Drugs 1988), but a small descriptive study suggested that injecting tends to persist, even if there are positive life changes (Battersby et al. 1992). We find that a gradual transition away from ampoules, using prescriptions including both forms, can be successful in less severe cases, and also that some individuals who cannot give up injecting completely can manage on a combination prescription which includes injectables on only one or two days of each week.

If injectables are used rather than the more routine methadone mixture, in our view the treatment contract must be correspondingly stricter. The abstinence from street drugs mentioned above is virtually mandatory, the principle being that if an individual persists in using additional drugs, he or she may not necessarily be discharged from treatment, but can do so on a routine mixture prescription rather than on one which has several disadvantages from our point of view, such as expense and the requirement for injection. There should be daily dispensing, whereas the pharmacy study by Strang et al. (1996) found that prescriptions for ampoules and tablets were actually less likely to be on this basis than those for mixture.

Ampoules come in various strengths, including 10 mg, 20 mg and 35 mg (all at 10 mg in 1 ml), and three 50 mg options, in 5 ml, 2 ml and 1 ml. The concentrated ampoules offer the benefit of less liquid for those who have difficulty in venous access, but the 50 mg in 1 ml in particular can cause troublesome stinging at the injection site. The ampoules are really intended for intramuscular injection, but in this indication it is accepted that drug misusers will use them intravenously where possible. Often peripheral veins cannot withstand this for long and the femoral vein will be used, for which services should give instruction.

The term 'needle fixation' is often used by patients and others, but the existence of this beyond an ordinary 'route preference' for drugs by injection is rare. Sometimes, users will describe toying around with needles and water to satisfy an urge, by way of backing up their claims to be on injectables, but the decision to prescribe should be based on sheer evidence of persistence of injecting over time, rather than on this rather dubious phenomenon.

### Case history

Michael is a 30-year-old man who has been a patient in our methadone clinic for three years. He has a ten-year history of opiate use in all, but previous treatment had been elsewhere on a detoxification basis. At one time he had strongly wished to come off drugs completely and went into a residential rehabilitation centre, but although he completed the stay satisfactorily he relapsed into heroin use soon afterwards. It is now agreed between us that his methadone treatment will need to continue for the foreseeable future.

On an established dose of 70 mg per day of methadone mixture Michael showed a good improvement, but it was clear he was not able to abstain completely from other drug use. He lives in an area where heroin and cocaine are both easily available, and these drugs regularly showed in his urine drug screens.

He considered heroin his main problem, strongly desiring the effect of that drug by injection. He could avoid this for a while, but the desire would build up and at least once a week he would need to have a 'fix'. After he had done this he would feel exasperated that he had spent money on drugs, with this causing particular problems between him and his girlfriend. He was strongly encouraged to adhere only to methadone, but we were reluctant to discharge him on the grounds of other drug use, since there had previously been exceptional social decline between periods of treatment.

After much discussion it was decided that Michael could have 70 mg of methadone in injectable form on one day per week, with methadone mixture on the other six days. On this combination it was required that all urine samples showed no other drugs, otherwise his treatment would revert to methadone mixture as previously. At first, appointments and urine sampling would be every two weeks, moving to monthly if there was good progress. Since this combination was instituted all Michael's urine tests have shown methadone only, and he is quite satisfied with this approach. He says that if he gets a strong desire to inject in the middle of the week, he knows that his injectable methadone is coming on Friday and this is enough to dissuade him from buying anything else. His girlfriend is equally impressed, and their relationship, and the wider ones with their families, have greatly improved. For the first time, however, he is beginning to have problems with his injection sites.

## Summary

Methadone is undoubtedly one of the most effective treatments we have in drug misuse. The systematic evidence from controlled and observational studies mostly relates to formalized methadone programmes characterized by daily attendance, supervised consumption of medication, compulsory counselling and structured social rehabilitation. Patients accepted into these early programmes typically had histories of several years of opiate dependence, failed rehabilitation attempts and marked social complications, and in the broader usage of methadone which has developed since, would undoubtedly be considered in the category of cases requiring long-term treatment. The highly impressive results of the formative studies can be considered partly due to this selection of severely dependent groups, and the exclusion of individuals with significant additional use of nonopiate drugs.

Over the years since methadone was introduced, patterns of drug misuse have changed greatly, and so has methadone treatment in many instances. There are now relatively few highly structured methadone programmes, particularly in Europe where there has been an emphasis on 'low-threshold' methadone treatment as a response to the HIV epidemic. In the 1980s, methadone prescribing was seen as one of the main strategies for reducing the transmission risks posed by injecting, along with needle exchange schemes and other harm-reduction measures. Partly on public health grounds, therefore, methadone was extended to a much wider population than previously, and policies shifted so that, for instance, users were retained in treatment even if abstinence from other drugs was not complete. Methadone treatment along these lines has been a pragmatic development, based on the assumption that prescribing at least readily reduces other drug use, and it has not been subjected to the same rigorous testing as the previous programmes. Indeed, there is often criticism of the harm-reduction model of prescribing, especially as it tends to be low dose, whereas the original investigators felt that high doses were required not only to relieve withdrawal symptoms and craving, but produce so-called narcotic blockade.

Two important reasons why modern methadone treatment tends to be lower dose are that the wider population of users are often using relatively small amounts of impure street heroin, and that, rightly or wrongly, there is often a desire on the part of those concerned for reduction and eventual abstinence. The purely medical model of methadone maintenance sees the drug as a necessary corrective treatment for the metabolic disorder of opiate dependence, a concept based on severely dependent individuals. In practice, many patients in current treatment wish to reduce their methadone over months or years, although such evidence as there is indicates that this is not often successful. The supporters of the current ways of methadone prescribing claim that it has led to a generally low rate of HIV in injecting drug users in the UK and elsewhere, and it is notable that the evidence for reduced HIV-risk behaviours and seroconversion rates does not all relate to rigid programmes. The high prevalence rates of hepatitis C which are now being demonstrated in injecting drug users suggest that harm-reduction measures in general have been much less successful in avoiding transmission of this more infective agent.

Partly because of the emphasis on HIV prevention, methadone prescribing presently constitutes an uneasy balance between individualized treatment, which aims for the best outcomes for each patient, and public health policy. Many patients in clinics are not definite maintenance candidates of the type originally envisaged, but rather drift into long-term treatment on broad harm-reduction grounds. The aims of treatment may be unclear in various ways, with also the paradoxical situation whereby a medical treatment is given to achieve substantially social benefits. A 'transparency of objectives' has been suggested where, if the main aim of treatment is to keep a drug misuser from re-offending or to improve his or her family relationships, then not only might treatment be funded by, say, probation services, but particular strategies may be required in terms of prescribed medication. The emphasis on retention in treatment has highlighted the fact that many drug misusers cannot adjust to the effects of methadone alone, and the social and other benefits might only accrue in some committed injectors or polydrug users if there is prescribing of injectable methadone, or additional or alternative medications.

Over the years there has gradually been less acceptance of the notion of methadone as a primary pharmacological treatment which normalizes the behaviour and personality of an addict, required in the way that insulin is required by a diabetic. This book sees methadone as a substitution treatment, being usually the clinically most suitable medication to employ in attempting to switch an individual from street drug use to a prescribed regime. The effects of methadone are very different from those of heroin, notably much less euphoriant, but many users value the stability that methadone brings, even though they may still be tempted to use other drugs at times. Given the basic nature of this treatment approach, which is not adopted in alcohol misuse or other forms of drug misuse, it is unsurprising that methadone produces powerful effects on attraction into treatment and patient retention, and overall reductions in many indicators of other drug misuse, ranging from injecting to social consequences. This is an invaluable option in a condition in which there are high relapse rates after detoxification, at least in established addicts, but inevitably there are also significant concerns about methadone. The ones which are primarily clinical issues, rather than broader social concerns, include the dominance of methadone patients in drug services at the expense of other types of drug misusers, the particular addictiveness of the drug, which is unimportant in outright maintenance treatment but which plagues attempts at reduction, and the specific side effects.

## 2

More than methadone? The case for other substitute drugs

### Introduction

For all the evidence in support of methadone, clinicians cannot fail to observe that not all dependent opiate misusers progress well on the treatment, even when it is made available over generous time scales. There may be any number of reasons for this to do with individual circumstances and clinical situations, but the nature and properties of the drug are also important. One problematic group are those users who appear to find it impossible to adjust to the noneuphoriant nature of methadone, desirable though that adjustment is generally considered to be. They will continue to use other drugs, often in direct combination with methadone, to gain some euphoria and so, as well as all the important considerations of motivation which such behaviour raises, the adequacy of the substitute drug must be called into question. If a maintenance methadone user persistently combines their drug with benzodiazepines, cocaine, cyclizine, or alcohol, ostensibly to make the effects more like those of heroin, it can be argued that fewer problems would result if heroin were actually prescribed, rendering the other drug-taking behaviours and risks unnecessary.

Most interest in this way has indeed focused on diamorphine, but other opiates have also been used with a similar rationale, and the first part of this chapter examines the relevant arguments and the limited available evidence. The subject arouses strong emotions, with some authorities finding it incomprehensible that anyone could apparently ignore the evidence for effectiveness of methadone, which is unparalleled in drug misuse treatment, to consider alternatives in any cases. Other clinicians pragmatically point out that, much though we may wish and encourage all patients to find methadone satisfactory, a substantial proportion of mainly long-term injectors manifestly cannot do so but retain some motivation for treatment, and that variations on the substitute prescribing theme can produce benefits in difficult cases.

The other types of situation in which methadone can seem an unsatisfactory substitution agent are towards the opposite end of the treatment spectrum. In uncomplicated maintenance treatment or for detoxification, the criticisms which are levelled at methadone relate not so much to the subjective effects, but to the aspects of addictiveness, abuse potential and toxicity. The issue of whether methadone is too addictive to be really suitable for detoxification is considered in detail in Chapter 3, and the controversial subject of methadone deaths in Chapter 7. Within this review of alternative opioids the particular claims are examined for buprenorphine, a drug which is both safer and less addictive than methadone, and which is being investigated in several countries.

The development of physical dependence on opiates before treatment is one of the main reasons why substitute prescribing is considered necessary and appropriate in this group of users. Such an approach is conventionally considered unsuitable in the case of other drug groups, but some clinicians argue that the principle can be applied with benefit to heavy amphetamine users. It is suggested that the distinction between physical and psychological dependence is scientifically unsatisfactory, that some heavy amphetamine users appear to closely resemble opiate users in their needs for treatment and harm-reduction measures, and that it is inequitable to deny this group an approach which has such an overwhelming effect on engagement in treatment. Some evidence from clinical experimentation with amphetamine prescribing is included in a general discussion here. The final section is a practical examination of the area of prescribing benzodiazepines to illicit drug users. Any such prescribing has inherent disadvantages and much potential for abuse, but in practice the situation arises extremely commonly, and a realistic appraisal of the issues and the limited appropriate indications is necessary.

## Diamorphine

Prescribing diamorphine for heroin users has attracted the most attention as an alternative maintenance approach including, inevitably, much coverage in the media. Its proponents claim, among other arguments, that giving the noneuphoriant methadone to individuals who are used to heroin almost invites the additional use of other drugs, as a 'high' will often still be sought. It is argued that, having gone down the route of substitute prescribing, it is more logical to give the pharmaceutical preparation of the preferred drug, rather than a drug that only approximates to its effects. Some critics advocate this as a general policy, but current clinical use in areas where diamorphine is available for this purpose tends to be limited to particular patient groups.

In the UK, diamorphine has been used for many years as one of the treatments of opiate misuse, and currently occupies a minority position alongside much more extensive prescribing of methadone. Methadone is given for the usual indication of dependent opiate misuse, and the vast majority of individuals in treatment will be encouraged to persist with this drug even when there are difficulties. Diamorphine is used by some clinicians in a proportion of long-term injectors who have failed to progress on oral or even injectable methadone, with very little prescribing of the drug outside this chronic, nearly always older group. The peripheral position of diamorphine within treatment was illustrated by a survey of the doctors who hold the Home Office licence which specialists can apply for to prescribe the drug (Sell et al. 1997). Forty-three doctors in the UK had such a licence, with the majority of those prescribing diamorphine only doing so for between one and ten individuals. This presumably represents a small fraction of those clinicians' total clinical caseloads and, in a short section for comments, enthusiasm for this option appeared somewhat lukewarm. Ratings of global outcome of diamorphine prescribing were mainly split between 'good' and 'average', with some clinicians stating that they only held a licence because diamorphine had been initiated by colleagues, or that they used the drug solely for short-term treatment. There was evidence of some more extensive usage, however, with three doctors prescribing for between 33 and 100 individuals.

Prescriptions issued for diamorphine in the UK have been analysed in a survey of drug misuse prescriptions at community pharmacies (Strang & Sheridan 1997a). One in every four pharmacies were included, and 64 ongoing heroin prescriptions were identified, constituting less than 2% of opiate prescriptions to addicts. Three-quarters of the prescriptions were for ampoules, but there was some use of tablets, liquid and cigarettes. Mean dosage was over three times the dosage for methadone prescriptions, with dispensing usually on a daily basis. Metrebian et al. (1996) have reviewed the subject from a clinical perspective, and provided some brief information from their own treatment service. In what the authors stated was the largest heroin prescribing clinic in the UK, 50 individuals were receiving the drug in doses ranging from 30 to 300 mg per day, as determined by tolerance testing. Most prescribing was in the form of ampoules, and the review discusses injectable prescribing in general.

It is well known that the tradition of some diamorphine prescribing in the UK relates to the so-called 'British System' of drug control (Strang & Gossop 1994). Legislation in the 1920s effectively placed the control of heroin and other addictive drugs in the hands of doctors to protect their use as medical treatments, and the subsequent response to illicit drug misuse included some maintenance treatment with the drug. Critics of current plans to investigate diamorphine prescribing claim that we already know what happens, from this previous experience in the 1960s and 1970s, and in this emotive area phrases like 'a giant leap back to the past' may be heard. Many clinicians feel that drug misuse is now so different in terms of subcultures and patterns of usage that a re-evaluation is indicated, but the results of the earlier controlled trial by Hartnoll et al. (1980) are nevertheless instructive. Ninety-six injecting heroin addicts requesting a diamorphine maintenance prescription were randomly allocated to treatment with injectable diamorphine or oral methadone for one year. Prescribing diamorphine did not substantially reduce use of street drugs, involvement with the drug subculture or even criminal activity, or produce greater improvement overall than methadone in general health and social functioning; with methadone treatment there was a polarized response, with some users progressing well but others having the worst outcomes, including more arrests. The fact, therefore, that some injectors made the transition satisfactorily to oral methadone, plus the limitation in benefits produced by diamorphine, would be seen by many as sufficient reason to support a conventional methadone policy but, as ever, it is the nonresponders who are the problem.

There has been much international interest recently in a project investigating heroin prescribing for drug misusers in Switzerland. The background and early results of the project, which also included prescribing intravenous methadone and morphine, have been described by Uchtenhagen et al. (1996). Methadone had been available in Switzerland since the late 1970s, but there was increasing public concern that drug misuse was becoming out of control, and it was apparent to the various authorities that large numbers of drug misusers had no interest in treatment as it currently stood. The present project was planned very much along harm-reduction lines, the main aim being to generally reduce HIV transmission risks by attracting previously reluctant users into treatment, and retaining them, with more acceptable prescriptions. The emphasis on retention was such that prescriptions would not be stopped on the basis of additional drug use, unless patient safety was compromised. Injecting of the medications was on-site, which eliminated diversion, and there were apparently no major problems with general acceptance of the project, for instance in neighbourhoods. In clinical terms, heroin proved not surprisingly to be the most desirable of the three drugs, but was only satisfactory in injectable form. The project included a cigarette preparation for those who had never injected, but testing showed much of the heroin to be destroyed in the burning process. Over the initial six months the retention rate of the project was 82%, and there were reported reductions in other drug use, illegal activities and prostitution, and general improvements in social stability and physical and psychological health. The authors aptly conclude that 'providing pharmaceutical heroin in this project permits to attract addicts who fail in multiple other treatment approaches and give them a new opportunity to take courage and engage in a therapeutic and rehabilitation programme without being forced to abstain from their preferred substance. It is not assured yet, however, to what extent positive changes in health and social status will continue over longer periods of time, and to what extent a drug-free lifestyle can be reached by participants in a later stage.' (Uchtenhagen et al. 1996). Further results from this sizeable study will add much to our knowledge of prescribing diamorphine and other injectable drugs.

We have noted the bias so far in the limited use of diamorphine prescribing towards long-term users, injectors and those who have failed on other treatments. This is due partly to the fact that the drug is most satisfactory in its injectable form, but also to the belief that oral methadone should be tried first, and that the euphoriant diamorphine would be inappropriate as a mainstream treatment. Patients on diamorphine in UK clinics tend to be those who have lobbied for the drug for many years, until the development of severe physical complications or another factor has additionally influenced the prescribing decision. A more radical view is that if methadone is widely perceived by drug misusers to be unsatisfactory, there should be consideration of diamorphine in those young users who are active in crime, have more acute family and social problems, and may be posing the most risks to the community. This would greatly disturb the balance of treatment as we currently have it, and it must be acknowledged that some of the strongest proponents of diamorphine prescribing partly base their views on the associated opinion that heroin should anyway be legalized (Marks 1996). In treatment settings we must primarily consider what produces benefit in the drug misusers we see, and on clinical grounds prescribing of diamorphine on any routine basis would simply seem to be unnecessary.

From a practical point of view, any expansion of the use of diamorphine to wider groups would mean investigation of smokable or oral preparations, to have alongside the injectable form. The smokable option has been advocated (Marks et al. 1991), but problems of bioavailability have not so far been overcome. Oral absorption is poor, but some patients appear to find the liquid preparation satisfactory, with daily dispensing especially required as this degrades quickly to morphine. Such options are of relevance not only for those who have never injected, but for long-term patients on injectable diamorphine or other injectable drugs who are unable to give up the enhanced subjective effects but who can no longer inject satisfactorily (although injected abuse of the liquid must be guarded against). The liquid preparation is preferable in the rare cases where diamorphine is used for detoxification instead of methadone, which may be done for reasons of patient acceptability or in an attempt to avoid methadone withdrawal symptoms (see Chapter 3).

All these uses remain uncommon at present in the UK even though it is fairly straightforward for specialists to gain the permission to prescribe diamorphine, and our clinic is typical of many in currently restricting its use to the kinds of severe patients referred to above. To merit a trial period on the drug, there must be specific risks caused by some form of additional drug taking and then monitoring in place to confirm that such usage stops when on diamorphine. When the drug has been used in this way, the most common general benefit claimed by patients is that they feel more energetic and better in mood than when on methadone. Like Uchtenhagen et al. (1996), we experience no major problem with combination prescriptions of injectable diamorphine and oral methadone, the methadone being used for its longer stabilizing effects after the effects of each day's diamorphine injections have worn off.

### Case history

Amanda is a 33-year-old woman whose case we inherited after she had been prescribed diamorphine in controversial circumstances. She had previously been a patient of the methadone clinic but her progress had generally been unsatisfactory, and eventually she had obtained treatment with diamorphine from a doctor in private practice. Unfortunately the doctor did not have the licence required to prescribe the drug, but by the time the situation was discovered treatment had been established for several months. It was agreed that we would take her back into our service, where diamorphine could be prescribed on a legal footing while her case was being reassessed.

Reviewing her history, it appeared that she had used heroin by injection for five years before being first prescribed methadone. She was from a relatively isolated small town where the limited network of users had few links with treatment services. She used heroin with her then husband, and both were eventually referred to the clinic after he had been charged with supplying the drug. They separated soon afterwards, and while he remained in treatment for only a short period, Amanda has been receiving prescribed medication since that time.

She never managed to stabilize on oral methadone, with virtually all urine samples showing morphine, benzodiazepines and/or amphetamine. She was prescribed benzodiazepines by her general practitioner, while she claimed to be unable to give up injecting heroin and she also drank alcohol quite heavily. Her methadone dose reached 120 mg per day, and for a short while before dropping out she was prescribed this in injectable form, but still she did not refrain from other drug use. She worked in a city department store, but her job was under threat because of frequent time off.

When she returned to the clinic following her period on diamorphine, she reported that she felt a prescription of that drug would be the answer to her difficulties. Because of her limited contacts with other users in treatment she did not actually grasp that this was a rare option, and she had been bemused by the problems of the legality of her prescription. She simply stated that she had 'never got on with methadone', claiming that it made her lethargic and depressed. She had particularly disliked the injectable form since it had damaged her veins more than street heroin ever had. On the grounds of obvious lack of progress with methadone it was agreed that we would prescribe injectable diamorphine, on a strict contract requiring absence of other drugs except benzodiazepines, which she now received on prescription in very small amounts. Her private prescription of diamorphine had in fact been inadequate, with a week's supply lasting only three days, and our own prescription was to be for 500 mg per day, with the contract enforced by two-weekly urine testing.

Although the circumstances of Amanda receiving diamorphine treatment have been unusual, her progress is now exemplary. All urine samples indicate diamorphine use only, with her finding no need to take even small amounts of benzodiazepines. She drinks alcohol no more than about once a month, on nights out with her work colleagues. She takes no street drugs, and her social, financial and work situations have improved greatly. She injects three times a day, with no problems in still using her arm veins. The only difficulty she has with treatment is in envisaging any alternative approach, and it is very unlikely that methadone will be able to be useful in future.

## Dipipanone (Diconal)

Diconal is a combination tablet of the opioid dipipanone, and cyclizine, the effects of which are highly regarded by drug users experienced with pharmaceutical opioids. Following widespread misuse of Diconal tablets by injection, in the UK in 1984 it was added to those drugs for which a licence is required for prescribing to addicts. The survey of doctors by Sell et al. (1997) found only 13 doctors to have a current licence, with as many prescribers considering the general outcome of prescribing Diconal to be 'poor', as 'good'. By any standards this would seem to have a very small place within the treatment spectrum, for use within specialist clinics for a minority of exceptional patients. An important feature of Diconal is that, like dextromoramide, it is much more euphoriant when injected than when taken orally, and so issuing tablets runs a high risk of misuse in this way.

## Cyclimorphine

Injectable Cyclimorphine ampoules contain either 10 mg or 15 mg of morphine, plus 50 mg of cyclizine. They are occasionally used as an injectable substitution treatment option for drug misusers, on two slightly different grounds.

The first usage is on the principle of providing an injectable substitute, of a more euphoriant nature, in the proportion of committed injectors for whom methadone in any form appears inadequate. As well as being antiemetic, cyclizine enhances the subjective effects of opiates, which would appear to partly account for the particular appeal of Diconal among drug misusers. Beyond injectable methadone therefore, Cyclimorphine may be more satisfying for some users in treatment and, the principle continues, may be more likely to enable abstinence from street drugs. This usage is therefore similar to that of diamorphine, and in the UK Cyclimorphine may sometimes be chosen where the doctor does not have the licence to prescribe diamorphine, or simply because of patient preference.

The other usage of Cyclimorphine occurs in areas where there is misuse of cyclizine tablets by injection (Ruben et al. 1989). This form of drug misuse, which is discussed in Chapter 4, causes severe behavioural disturbances and physical complications, and some clinicians attempt to prevent excessive misuse of the crushed tablets by prescribing a controlled amount of cyclizine in Cyclimorphine. This could clearly only be suitable for those who misuse cyclizine along with injected opiates, but this appears to be the usual combination. Certainly, giving methadone tablets to cyclizine misusers is particularly inadvisable, as it seems that universally both drugs will be crushed and used together. The great disadvantage of prescribing Cyclimorphine in these circumstances is that urine screening cannot detect whether only prescribed cyclizine or street supplies are being used, and assessment of progress relies largely on general clinical impression. Given the adverse effects of cyclizine, and the risks of diversion in areas where cyclizine is a highly prized drug, the prescribing of Cyclimorphine (or cyclizine ampoules) to attempt to counter cyclizine misuse appears an unsatisfactory approach, even given the absence of other useful treatment options.

Cyclimorphine can be considered next down from diamorphine in the hierarchy of euphoriant opioids which may be given as treatment and, as with that drug, if it is prescribed in very rare cases rather than methadone, treatment contracts must be correspondingly strict.

## Morphine

Because diamorphine is converted to morphine in the body, prescribing the two drugs may be considered broadly similar. However, the initial subjective effects of diamorphine are crucial, and morphine is inherently a much less attractive proposition. In the trial of injectable drugs in Switzerland (Uchtenhagen et al. 1996), in which the morphine protocol was based on previous experience in the Netherlands, two of the morphine prescribing groups were curtailed because of poor acceptability by participants. Of side effects, histamine-like reactions on intravenous injection were most frequently reported.

Some patients on methadone mixture claim that, of oral preparations, they feel better on morphine, usually in terms of energy and mood. Of the adverse effects of methadone, weight gain, sweating and reduced libido may also be less problematic with morphine, and Fischer et al. (1996) have reported high acceptability of morphine in this way, with the results of treatment being as good as with methadone. Tablet preparations are available in slow-release forms, although where there is concern about risk of abuse by injection morphine sulphate mixture may be used. There are plans to introduce a combination tablet containing naloxone, which is a deterrent to injected misuse as the naloxone would be active intravenously but not orally, and so injection would precipitate withdrawal. This approach is discussed in more detail in the section below on buprenorphine, for which drug the development of a similar combination product is further advanced, although for pharmacological reasons the combination of naloxone with morphine may be more satisfactory. Two general disadvantages of morphine treatment are that it is more expensive than methadone, and that on urine testing it may be impossible to distinguish the prescribed drug from morphine as the excreted metabolite of heroin, unless the specific heroin metabolite 6–monoacetyl morphine is detected.

### Case history

Alan is a 32-year-old man with a 16-year history of opiate dependence. His formative years of drug taking were spent not in using street heroin, but pharmaceutical opioids obtained from robberies of chemists premises. In this way he would inject Diconal, dextromoramide, morphine and diamorphine ampoules, and a wide range of other drugs. He joked with us once that methadone was always the last to be used of any raided supplies because of its boring effects. He had had several prison sentences, and any contact with treatment services was usually short-lived.

In the past five years Alan has made a great effort to move away from the criminal lifestyle and illicit drug taking. He has been helped in this by his relationship with his girlfriend, who is from a very different background and supports them both with a full-time job. He has become a patient of our methadone clinic, and at his appointments they both emphasize their determination that he should have nothing to do with nonprescribed drug use. His lifestyle has become extremely restricted, but his main objective has been to avoid any activities which might lead to further legal problems or imprisonment.

Very early in his treatment it was apparent that long-term substitution medication would be needed, and he was initially maintained on methadone mixture 70 mg per day. His requirement proved much more than this and, in increments, the dosage increased to 150 mg per day. He reported no major problems in stopping injecting, and superficially his progress appeared reasonable. He was no longer involved in crime, and his urine drug screens showed only benzodiazepines in addition to methadone. He was obtaining these from various contacts, and in due course it was decided that we instead should prescribe him small amounts of diazepam and nitrazepam under controlled conditions.

Closer examination revealed a situation which was far from satisfactory. Apart from going to the chemist each day to collect his medication, Alan barely left the house, and his girlfriend reported that he had no interest in any activities. He was taciturn and depressed, had little energy and had become significantly overweight. He was avoiding other drugs but this appeared to be a daily battle, in which he was preoccupied with the lack of any discernable subjective effect from his methadone. It was not considered that he was under-medicated, since with or without benzodiazepines he usually appeared mildly sedated with slightly slurred speech. When pressed about his difficulties Alan gave the impression of being intensely frustrated, and the obvious conclusion was that, even after years of trying, he had failed to adjust satisfactorily to methadone's limited effects.

It was felt that a trial period was indicated on an alternative oral substitute medication which would present no risk of abuse by injection. Morphine sulphate liquid was prescribed, in a dose correspondingly higher than methadone due to the shorter half-life. Benzodiazepine dosages were reduced as part of the agreement. After three months there has been a limited, but significant, improvement in Alan's condition overall. Although his weight has not decreased he has more energy and interest, so that he helps in doing some jobs around the house. He is apparently never intoxicated, but feels some satisfaction from the morphine effect in the early stages after his doses, and there has been a general improvement in mood. No disadvantage is apparent in taking morphine, and this is to be continued.

## Issues in prescribing euphoriant opioids

All the above drugs have been discussed as possible substitute treatments which are more euphoriant than methadone. The evidence relating to their use is minimal in comparison to that for methadone, and they seem likely for the time being to remain peripheral possibilities for a minority of patients in particular circumstances. The euphoriant properties have been identified as a rationale for treatment, and this has various implications both for the individuals concerned, and in terms of overall treatment within a clinic.

At an individual level, the issues are similar to those which arise in giving injectable methadone (see page 44). Unless routine usage is contemplated, there is no way around the fact that, in terms of general progress, users have to 'fail' at methadone treatment to be considered for diamorphine, Cyclimorphine or an alternative opioid. Also, a recurring theme in the discussions of alternative prescribing, whether it be additional benzodiazepines, injectables or euphoriant medications, is that the potential *disadvantages* are such that some major *advantage* needs to accrue if it is done, that usually being complete abstinence from street drugs as identified in a strict treatment contract. The nature of the more euphoriant treatments makes it very important that security must be higher, including daily dispensing to avoid over-use; unfortunately the opposite can sometimes happen when a user, successful in securing an alternative treatment, persuades the doctor that he or she is experienced enough to manage less frequent collection. Prescribers should also acknowledge that giving injectables or diamorphine tends to be 'one-way traffic', with the policy difficult to retract once established. This may not matter in the context of definite maintenance treatment, and indeed the situation is not inevitable as some users do find the euphoriant prescription which they have been seeking too destabilizing once it is actually available, and wish to revert to methadone.

The prescribing of alternative opioids may cause wider problems within a clinic population. Once it is known that they are given in some cases, individuals who are basically making good progress in adjusting to methadone may nevertheless be tempted to seek a more euphoriant medication. Even if they do not actually do this, there may be some unease if they see those who are making less progress 'rewarded' with alternative drugs. This, of course, begs the whole question of whether most patients are or are not seeking to make the various changes away from their previous types of drug use, but my own experience is that the availability of different prescriptions for some within a clinic does not lead to unmanageable and unwarranted levels of demand. In Sheffield, where we use the more euphoriant medications in some cases, although many patients experience common problems relating to the use of methadone, the number of requests for alternatives is not high.

Our clinic in North Nottinghamshire is more typical of many in the UK which choose to make only methadone available, of the opiate substitution treatments. While this can be considered appropriate simply in terms of the supporting evidence, it also reflects a difference which is often found between clinics in smaller towns and large cities. Our two services and the layout of services in general are discussed in Chapter 5, but there is still a legacy of the recommendations of the Advisory Council on the Misuse of Drugs (1982), whereby services treating more severe cases are to be found in the main cities. These can receive referrals from the other more localized services and so have concentrations of individuals who have not responded to standard treatment, while arguably it might also be anticipated that wider prescribing responses are required for city populations, where there are generally higher levels of drug availability, associated social problems and individual drug usage. Whether that is valid or not, it works well in practice for many services to limit their prescribing tariff and to refer exceptional cases onto a separate service with alternative protocols. As described in the chapter on services, however, changes in the National Health Service mean that referral between treatment centres is actually becoming more difficult, and so there is increasingly a requirement for service providers in individual areas to offer all the treatments which they consider to be necessary.

## Levo-alpha-acetylmethadol (LAAM)

LAAM is emerging as a potentially important alternative substitution agent in the treatment of opiate dependence (Ling et al. 1994, Eissenberg et al. 1997). It is an opioid agonist with basically similar properties to methadone although it is not, strictly speaking, a form of that drug. It is the metabolites of LAAM rather than the drug itself which are active, and the major difference compared to methadone is that there is a much longer duration of action, up to 72 hours. In maintenance treatment LAAM therefore need only be taken on three days per week, as opposed to the daily dosing with methadone.

The interest which clinicians will have in LAAM depends largely on their current policy arrangements for the dispensing of methadone. In clinics where there is no take-home medication policy and methadone patients have to attend daily for supervised consumption, a reduction in dosing to three times per week could clearly have great advantages both for patients and for the services. Ling et al. (1994) point to patients being more involved in nondrug activities, more efficient use of staff time and reductions in expense, less need for special 'privileges' such as allowing a methadone patient to miss one day's attendance, and advantages for neighbourhoods in which clinics are sited. In the UK at present there is less immediate relevance, as most arrangements are for patients to collect methadone at community pharmacies, and daily dispensing is not often required. However, the general policy climate is moving towards more secure treatment (see Chapter 7), and also many clinics are having to consider on-site dispensing on expense and other grounds, and so LAAM should prove of increasing interest as it becomes available for clinical use. Direct clinical advantages of LAAM are that it provides a particularly stabilizing drug effect with little daily fluctuation, and that because of its relatively slow onset of action it is less likely than other medications to be abused by injection.

The motivation of patients is likely to be an issue in relation to the properties of LAAM, as candidates need to have progressed beyond the stage of seeking any short-term drug effect, or psychologically requiring to take a drug at frequent intervals. These changes are inherent in methadone treatment, but LAAM can be seen as taking them each one step further. Another reason for selecting relatively well-motivated patients to receive LAAM is that diversion of prescribed supplies of the drug is particularly undesirable. The long duration of action means that some overdose situations, with or without other drugs, could be especially dangerous, and supervised consumption is likely to be recommended in all settings to reduce such risks.

In the USA the implementation of LAAM treatment within clinics has been much slower than anticipated. Rawson et al. (1998) have examined the reasons in detail, observing that the ever-increasing demands in terms of safety and efficacy trials and regulatory procedures have been more significant in the delay than any problems actually to do with the drug. Private methadone programmes in which the requirement for daily attendance is linked to profits have been reluctant to transfer to LAAM, although so have programmes which do not require frequent attendance, i.e. the situation analogous to the common one in the UK. The authors feel that important lessons have been learnt for the introduction of future new medications for drug misuse in the USA, but they reinforce the potential clinical benefits of LAAM.

## Buprenorphine

The properties of buprenorphine make it another interesting candidate as a treatment drug. Basically it can be seen as a substitution treatment, but it is a mixed opiate agonist–antagonist, so that it relieves withdrawal symptoms but partly blocks other opiates, has limited reinforcing effects and is safe in overdosage. The drug is used as an analgesic in the form of 0.2 mg and 0.4 mg Temgesic tablets, which are taken sublingually, as there is poor oral bioavailability. As a treatment for opiate misuse the dose required appears to lie between 2 and 16 mg per day (Johnson et al. 1995, Ling et al. 1998) – Strain et al. (1994a) found an optimum of 8.9 mg per day – and so 2 mg and 8 mg tablets have been made for research and clinical use. Buprenorphine is long-acting and so it can be taken daily, or in larger doses spaced further apart (Amass et al. 1994). In comparison with methadone, the drug has four main possible advantages, as indicated in Table 2.1.

Research evidence is accumulating on this combination of features, which all relate to the agonist–antagonist activity of the drug. It seems impossible to die from overdose of buprenorphine alone because of a ceiling on agonist effects (Walsh et al. 1994), although a combination with other drugs such as benzodiazepines can be fatal (Reynaud et al. 1998). The subjective effects are less reinforcing than those of methadone, and withdrawal symptoms are milder (Bickel & Amass 1995). Although use in pregnancy has been limited, it has been generally unproblematic and there appears to be a correspondingly low level of neonatal withdrawal

Table 2.1. *Possible advantages of buprenorphine over methadone as substitution treatment in opiate misuse*

| |
|---|
| Safer |
| Less addictive |
| Less interaction with other euphoriant drugs |
| Quicker transfer to naltrexone after detoxification |

features (Reisinger 1997). The limitation in agonist effects produces less interaction with other euphoriant drugs, so that there is a possible advantage in the problematic situation when opioid-maintained patients combine their drug with cocaine for a 'speedball' effect (Foltin & Fischman 1996). Finally, after detoxification with buprenorphine the opiate antagonist naltrexone can be started for relapse prevention much sooner than it can after methadone, possibly as little as one day after completion (Rosen & Kosten 1995).

The theoretical basis for buprenorphine treatment is therefore strong, and the evidence from the research centres, mainly in the USA, is encouraging, but how will the drug fare in wider clinical practice? It has recently been launched in France where, interestingly, substitution treatment with methadone was only generally recommended at around the same time, the emphasis having previously been firmly on psychological treatment. The early results of trials of buprenorphine in detoxification and maintenance treatment, there and in other European countries, have been reviewed by Chapleo et al. (1997), and are mainly promising. However, some problems were noted in Denmark which, continuing the theme we have discussed in this chapter, reflect buprenorphine's position as an even *less* euphoriant treatment option than methadone: some patients dropped out of a maintenance phase because they felt 'too normal' and requested a return to methadone, others continued to inject heroin (although apparently without euphoriant effect), and additional benzodiazepine use was common, apparently because this did enhance the subjective effects. Once again, therefore, it seems that the ability of individuals to accept a noneuphoriant effect of the substitute drug determines their progress in treatment, and in the future we may be weighing the various advantages of buprenorphine against only a moderate proportion achieving this, depending on patient selection.

In the UK we have a particular apprehension about buprenorphine, as for many years injected buprenorphine tablets were one of the main drugs of misuse in some of our cities (Lavelle et al. 1991). An ingenious method has been devised by the manufacturers aimed at countering misuse by injection, in the form of a combination tablet of buprenorphine and naloxone (Chapleo & Walter 1997). The theory is that as naloxone is ineffective sublingually it will not interfere with the buprenorphine if the combination tablet is properly taken by that route, but if the tablet is abused by injection the effect of the naloxone will be experienced, and withdrawal precipitated. This appears a very interesting prospect for use in areas where there is a history of buprenorphine injecting, but at this stage further evidence is required as to exactly how ineffective naloxone is by the sublingual route, and also the extent to which it does in fact displace buprenorphine from opiate receptors. It could be that the lack of interference by naloxone in sublingual usage is because the latter effect is not strong, which would leave open the possibility of 'successful' intravenous abuse of the combination tablet. It seems likely that an individual using heroin who injected the tablet would experience immediate withdrawal due to the more rapid binding of naloxone than buprenorphine, but quite what the adverse effects would be if a habitual buprenorphine user injected the combination preparation remains to be clarified.

The use of buprenorphine as a detoxification treatment is also discussed in Chapter 3.

## Dihydrocodeine

In services which aim to offer a range of prescribing options, dihydrocodeine has some appeal as a relatively minor opioid which produces less dependence than methadone. As such it may be seen as bridging the gap in treatments between methadone and the purely nonsubstitute detoxification options, such as lofexidine. Many clinicians, however, have a mainly negative view of this drug, due to the uncontrolled usage which frequently occurs when drug misusers obtain it from general practitioners, which is easily done on various grounds.

In the North Nottinghamshire service, where we carry out a lot of community detoxifications, we offer dihydrocodeine and additional symptomatic medication as one of our treatment options. This is a set reducing course over 7–14 days, which is prescribed in exact instalments to avoid erratic usage (see page 86 and Appendix 1). Long-term prescribing with dihydrocodeine is generally considered unsuitable, although clinically some patients are encountered who use an ongoing low dose in a stable way in preference to methadone, and it is perhaps questionable to insist on the more addictive methadone in such circumstances. An exceptionally favourable report of dihydrocodeine prescribing to drug misusers was by MacLeod et al. (1998), who audited the progress of 200 patients in substitution treatment over several years. The setting was a general practice in Edinburgh which specializes in drug misuse treatment and works closely with a drug counselling service; with dihydrocodeine prescribed more frequently than methadone for opiate misusers, there were no major differences between patients on the two medications in retention in treatment, death rate and behaviour change. Similarly positive results were reported in relation to maintenance with codeine or dihydrocodeine in Germany (Krausz et al. 1998), in which country long-term methadone treatment is relatively rarely used.

In terms of relative potency, a 30 mg dihydrocodeine tablet is equivalent to 3 mg of methadone, but, in practice, higher dosing with dihydrocodeine is required because of its shorter half-life. Slow-release tablets are also available, with therefore an increased apparent half-life. These are not particularly suitable for detoxification courses, where there are frequent reductions in dosage, but may be useful in those cases where ongoing treatment at a stable dosage is accommodated.

## Amphetamines

As indicated at the start of the chapter, there is some support for the view that the model of substitute prescribing which is used for opiate misusers should be extended to users of amphetamine. The availability of methadone enables treatment to be much more realistic by avoiding the requirement to be completely free of all opioid drugs, and the restriction of such an approach to users of one drug type can be viewed as both artificial and inequitable. The positive effect of methadone on attraction into treatment is obvious, and it is argued that this effect is particularly needed in amphetamine users, who are generally a younger group but who are at significant risk of major psychiatric and physical complications (Klee 1992). In the UK amphetamine use is extremely common, and it is mainly the HIV harm-reduction agenda which has produced calls for a look at prescribing amphetamines, although not any other nonopiate drugs. So how suitable is it to offer such an option?

There are proportionately far more occasional and recreational users of amphetamine than of heroin, and so it would seem only relevant to apply the prescribing parallel at the heavier end of amphetamine usage. Even so, the conventional view is that since amphetamine is not a drug of true physical dependence, there is not the same requirement to intervene with a substitute to break the cycle whereby a drug is taken to avoid withdrawal symptoms. (The contrary view is that the emphasis on physical, meaning bodily, symptoms is unsatisfactory now that we appreciate the neurochemical basis for so-called psychological withdrawal features.) Also conventionally, amphetamine is seen as an inherently more destabilizing drug, with its stimulant effect and risk of psychosis, so with these properties it is not suitable to prescribe. Even if those objections are overcome, there is not a form of amphetamine which is long acting, one of the benefits of methadone for heroin users. Nevertheless, the contrast between treatment received by opiate and amphetamine users is stark, and the success of methadone, at least in engaging drug misusers, is such that an increasing number of clinicians are attracted to some experimentation with amphetamine prescribing. Certainly in clinical practice one encounters some daily users of large amounts of injected amphetamine who appear dependent in any meaningful sense of the word, and have the adverse social consequences which effectively represent much of the rationale for prescribing a substitute to heroin users. It is notable that such users typically do not appear excessively stimulated by amphetamine, but rather they are agitated at times of withdrawal, as if a paradoxical effect may be at work.

Fleming & Roberts (1994) reported the results of a small-scale experiment with amphetamine prescribing over three years in a UK clinic. Acceptance criteria included at least six months' daily injecting of the drug, and subjects received 30 mg of dexamphetamine sulphate per day in liquid form. The prescribed courses did not necessarily reduce, with two-thirds of the total subjects still receiving prescriptions at the time of reporting, at a mean duration of 15 months. Medication consumption was supervised, and there were compulsory group meetings aimed at enhancing motivation and advising on harm reduction. With this approach over half the subjects were apparently able to stop injecting, as confirmed by physical examination, and there were substantial reductions in injecting by the remainder. There were consequent reductions in HIV-risk behaviours, although sexual practices were largely unchanged. The anticipated increase in amphetamine users presenting for treatment did occur. The authors observed that their results might have been even better had they prescribed higher doses of dexamphetamine; their calculation, which took into account the very low purity and presence of active and inactive forms in street amphetamine, was based on a street usage of 1 g per day, but probably most daily injectors use more than that.

A report of similar treatment has come from Victoria, Australia, also with encouraging results (Sherman 1990). A group of 14 street amphetamine addicts, mostly injectors, were prescribed 20–90 mg of dexamphetamine sulphate per day, with a substance administered to alkalinize the urine to prolong the half-life of the drug. Stabilization followed by slow reduction was the aim and, although treatment became prolonged in some cases, others apparently remained drug-free after their reducing course. As with many areas of experimental prescribing, however, most experience has been in the UK, where the extent to which this option has been tried is perhaps surprising in that it goes against very clear advisory guidance. Guidelines on clinical management of drug misuse issued by the Department of Health to all doctors (Department of Health 1991) stated simply that 'it is undesirable to prescribe substitute stimulant drugs as the risk of them being misused is very high'. Nevertheless, at a time when those were the current guidelines, Strang & Sheridan (1997b) estimated from a survey of community pharmacies that approximately a thousand addicts were receiving amphetamine prescriptions. Only 8% of prescriptions were from private practice, and nearly half were from general practitioners.

The views and clinical practice of drug misuse specialists in the UK in relation to amphetamine prescribing were also surveyed in the same period (Bradbeer et al. 1998) with, remarkably, 60% of 149 respondents considering that this approach had a place in clinical management. Forty-six per cent of the responding specialists did actually prescribe amphetamine, with others who approved in principle, but did not do so, giving lack of experience or budget limitations as their reasons. The main reasons for not approving of prescribing were a lack of evidence to say that it helps, risk of psychosis, no physical addiction, and budget limitations. The survey included some details of prescribing policies, and Table 2.2 indicates the features which emerged as something of a consensus.

Prescribing was mainly considered for long-term amphetamine injectors, and half the respondents also required absence of mental illness as a criterion. Dexamphetamine sulphate tablets were prescribed more than the suspension, at a mean maximum dose of 66 mg per day, while one clinician was using injectable amphetamine ampoules. Two-thirds of prescribers did not set a time limit on the period for which individuals could receive prescriptions, with monitoring apparently nearly always by urine screening and examination of injection sites. In practice, the latter is particularly useful in this group, as the committed long-term injectors for whom prescribing is considered are typically reluctant to use street

Table 2.2. *Features of amphetamine*
*prescribing by drug misuse specialists in the*
*UK*

| |
|---|
| *Criteria* |
| Long-term use |
| Injecting |
| No mental illness |
| *Prescription* |
| Dexamphetamine tablets or suspension |
| 20–200 mg/day |
| Not time-limited |
| *Monitoring* |
| Urine |
| Injection sites |
| *Location* |
| More outside London |

Based on Bradbeer et al. (1998)

amphetamine in any other way. Also, a special urinalysis technique has been described which largely enables separate identification of prescribed dexamphetamine and street amphetamine, by measuring the isomer ratio of $d$-amphetamine, which is present in both, to $l$-amphetamine, which is in the street preparation only (Tetlow & Merrill 1996).

It seems therefore that there is quite a widespread willingness in the UK to experiment with amphetamine prescribing, presumably by extension from the experience with methadone. Some of the general practitioners who prescribe may perhaps be those who work closely with community drug teams, and have been influenced by their policy arguments. Strang & Sheridan (1997b), however, are concerned both by the extent of amphetamine prescribing in the absence of good supporting evidence, and by the relative infrequency of daily dispensing and general lack of safeguards against diversion. They regret 'the lack of coherence of a national treatment response in which such extensive amphetamine prescribing could have developed largely uncharted', and point out that 'if the development of health care is, in future, to be more evidence-based, then new evidence-based guidance to specialist and general practitioners will be required'. This would seem to be a classic area in which there is tension between the principle of waiting for firm evidence from controlled studies, notoriously difficult to do in drug misusers, and some appeal of the policy arguments for engaging and providing active clinical intervention for this group. Most clinicians involved with amphetamine prescribing would agree that the treatment is not going to be in the same league as methadone, but they probably also have some cases who have derived substantial clinical benefit. The security aspects of prescribing are not fundamentally different from those for methadone, although daily dispensing of amphetamine is made much more difficult in the UK by the fact that the drug cannot be prescribed on the specialist multiple-dispensing controlled drug forms.

Where services have a policy of restricting amphetamine prescribing to short reducing courses, this often seems to have more to do with the uncertain basis for this form of treatment, and the risk of adverse effects, than any strong expectation that abstinence can be readily achieved. The risks of psychosis and mood disturbance are sometimes perceived to be higher with prescribed dexamphetamine than street amphetamine, and even in cases where the general harm-reduction benefits of prescribing have come about, long-term continuation may be considered inadvisable. In some cases, however, individuals appear to require only a short 'detoxification', in which case reductions may be achieved either by cuts in daily dosage, or by progressively omitting days in a week from the prescription, therefore mimicking recreational usage. At the heavy end of the scale, although the limited study evidence includes some good results in reducing injecting, there may be a group of committed injectors who do not respond favourably to oral dexamphetamine. There have been some attempts to use injectable methylamphetamine, the rationale being similar to that for injectable methadone, but in a previous era this was considered unsuccessful (Hawkes et al. 1969). Given the lack of overall evidence to support amphetamine prescribing this would seem to be an experiment too far and, with tablets liable to be crushed and injected, limited prescribing attempts should probably be restricted to dexamphetamine sulphate liquid at the present time.

### Case history

Peter is 46 years old, married with two children. He has been using amphetamines for 30 years, starting at a time when pharmaceutical amphetamines and barbiturates were prominent in the illicit drug scene, at nightclubs. In the early years he also abused pharmaceutical opioids, and he has continued to have cannabis and alcohol regularly. He went through a period of undoubted alcohol dependence, but throughout his 'career' his favoured drug has been amphetamine.

Following earlier occasional contacts Peter was referred to our service a year ago, largely as a result of his wife's concerns. Both she and Peter felt that a lifestyle change was required, and that the needs of their teenage children were being neglected. Peter's usage of amphetamine had gradually increased to about 7 g per day, injecting about six times per 24 hours. After each injection he would go to his bedroom and listen to loud 'rave' music for hours, and his wife was exasperated that he generally did very little else. Some evenings he would also go on to nightclubs, where he would use ecstasy.

Treatment aimed at short-term cessation of amphetamine use was considered completely unrealistic. After the necessary discussions the substitution prescribing option was initiated, with the harm-reduction objective of at least reducing Peter's injecting and use of street amphetamine. He was given dexamphetamine sulphate liquid 60 mg per day, with a plan to reduce gradually over the following months.

Treatment has been very successful, with a remarkable change in Peter's behaviour. Regular examination of injecting sites confirms his and his wife's reports of a dramatic decline in street amphetamine use, with many benefits for their domestic situation. Finances have greatly improved, the children's needs are being attended to, and they are to take a family holiday. Peter's behaviour is generally much more appropriate, and for the first time in years he is helping his wife in house duties. Although he had not been prone to psychosis, he had previously had much mood disturbance on street amphetamine, and his mood state has also greatly improved.

Because of the benefits we have not imposed a rapid reduction, with just two incremental reductions to 50 mg per day. However, we have gradually introduced amphetamine-free days, and his prescription is now for only three days each week.

## Benzodiazepines

The issues relating to benzodiazepine prescribing in polydrug users are somewhat different from those considered so far in this chapter, partly because benzodiazepine misuse is usually a secondary or peripheral form of drug usage. As a starting point, it can be observed that the only situation in which it is definitely advisable to prescribe benzodiazepines to an illicit drug user is that of short-term withdrawal from benzodiazepine misuse, where there is demonstrable physical dependence, and within a closely monitored arrangement. We also find it virtually essential to include benzodiazepines as symptomatic treatment in our quick opiate detoxification regimes such as that primarily using lofexidine (see Chapter 3), but in many other instances prescribing benzodiazepines carries a risk of erratic or even dangerous usage. Clearly, a large proportion of the benzodiazepines in the illicit drug scene come from diverted prescribed supplies, and the relatively easy availability of benzodiazepines, prescribed or nonprescribed, is extensively exploited by drug misusers. In the treatment setting, an approach of prescribing benzodiazepines to some methadone patients has its proponents, but also inherent disadvantages. Various situations in which prescribing arises will be considered in turn.

### Detoxification from benzodiazepine misuse

In this indication, the most important clinical consideration is determining what level of treatment is required. The answer seems to be, not as much as might be expected from the evidence relating to ordinary low-dose usage. Since it was demonstrated that physical dependence on benzodiazepines could occur in a proportion of cases (Tyrer et al. 1981), individuals who have become dependent after prescription for minor psychiatric disorders are typically offered reducing courses of benzodiazepines lasting several months or more (Lader & Morton 1991). To adopt the equivalent approach in drug misusers, with conversions for the far higher dosages that many of this group consume, would be quite unmanageable and inadvisable, and the first reason to avoid this is that not all benzodiazepine misusers become physically dependent. We demonstrated (Seivewright & Dougal 1993) that polydrug users in situations of stopping benzodiazepines can experience classical benzodiazepine withdrawal symptoms, in our study more severe after high dosage, multiple benzodiazepine use, and oral rather than injected use. With regard to the *proportion* of polydrug users who develop such symptoms, Williams et al. (1996) found in a detoxification unit that benzodiazepine withdrawal symptoms emerged in less than half of opiate addicts reporting current benzodiazepine misuse. Furthermore, in that study the dose of diazepam required for stabilization in those who did exhibit withdrawal features was unrelated to claimed previous benzodiazepine usage, at a mean dose of 40 mg per day.

This low level of prescribing is supported by the findings of Harrison et al. (1984), that in 23 individuals who had previously used a mean diazepam equivalent of 140 mg per day, diazepam detoxification starting at 40% of reported daily consumption, followed by daily tapering by 10%, ensured satisfactory completion in most cases. Also, a reduction from

60 mg of diazepam over six days has specifically been claimed to avoid convulsions in benzodiazepine misusers who had previously had that complication (Scott 1990). Even in individuals who do require treatment, therefore, it appears that relatively low-dose short benzodiazepine detoxification courses are adequate, which is to be welcomed given the difficulties which would otherwise be presented, and the misuse potential of prescribed medication. In terms of alternatives, there are case reports of carbamazepine being effective in withdrawal from up to 1000 mg of diazepam equivalent per day (Ries et al. 1989), but the extent to which that drug may be suitable as a withdrawal treatment in benzodiazepine misuse is unclear, particularly for community treatment.

**Other benzodiazepine prescribing**

A huge amount of unsatisfactory prescribing of benzodiazepines to drug misusers is encountered, including situations where they appear to be given as little more than a token gesture, to provide some satisfaction without the complications of issuing specific treatments such as methadone. Guidance on such matters is an important role for drug services, and also the precedents set by our own prescribing must always be borne in mind. Although in various situations we may see a case for some prescribing of benzodiazepines, any such prescribing to polydrug users can make it more difficult for us to advise others not to do this.

One emerging usage of short-term benzodiazepines is in states characterized by agitation, such as withdrawal states in stimulant users. In a survey of treatment of cocaine misuse in England, we found that over 10% of services had recently prescribed benzodiazepines to primary cocaine users, in a range of clinical situations (Donmall et al. 1995). Withdrawal from heavy use of crack cocaine provides a good example of the need to weigh the possible benefits of benzodiazepines in reducing agitation and withdrawal distress against the risk of erratic usage in an unstable situation, and the problems of establishing a precedent, including sometimes introducing a user to a new medication of misuse. There is also the concern that benzodiazepines may paradoxically increase aggressiveness, a phenomenon which is often quoted although the actual evidence is not strong (Bond 1993). This is potentially important in drug misusers, who as a group have high rates of aggressive and impulsive behaviours, but there is a suggestion from animal experiments with benzodiazepines that the aggression-enhancing effect occurs in those whose basal levels are relatively low (Mos & Oliver 1987).

## Case history

Carl is a 25-year-old man who was referred urgently and presented to the clinic along with his mother. He had been using crack cocaine for two years, and it was apparent that he had previously been a dealer in this drug. This was in the context of a generally criminal lifestyle, with previous convictions for armed robbery. He said that when initially dealing in the drug he 'never touched it myself', but that now he had a substantial crack habit. He used the drug compulsively with extreme craving, and gave the example of obtaining a financial loan to buy a car and then spending all the money in two days on crack. A urine drug screen confirmed use of cocaine, and there was evidence of related instability of mood, with Carl breaking down in tears in the assessment appointments. His mother was extremely distressed and told us that Carl had stolen and sold most of the valuable family possessions.

Residential treatment appeared the only likely way of making an impact on Carl's crack cocaine use, and plans were made for an admission. This could not happen immediately, and in the meantime Carl was prescribed fluoxetine 20 mg per day, and diazepam 20–30 mg per day. He was keen to try to withdraw himself from crack without going into hospital, and he and his mother were instructed about his use of the two medications. They were advised that diazepam would reduce anxiety and agitation, and might help relieve craving for crack.

One week later Carl told us that he had managed to completely avoid crack use, which was supported by urine sampling. His mother said that he had appeared drowsy on the diazepam, a medication which he had not had before, while Carl reported a generally helpful calming effect. He had also taken the fluoxetine, and there was a suggestion of a reduction in depression. After another week the situation was similar, although with the sedative effects of diazepam less marked. Carl felt that he did not need inpatient treatment as he had been able to stop using crack in this way, but unfortunately after that he dropped out of outpatient contact with us.

Benzodiazepines obtained by illicit drug users are no doubt put to a range of uses, of varying drug-related harm. The implications of controlled usage in opiate misusers in treatment are considered below, and in the discussions on opiate detoxification. Gossop et al. (1991) found that addicts in opiate withdrawal treatment had frequently used benzodiazepines in attempts at self-detoxification; this may arguably be seen as constructive use, but it may have been very uncontrolled and, given the setting, the attempts had clearly not been ultimately successful. Benzodiazepines appear to provide nonspecific relief in withdrawal from virtually any drug, including opiates (Drummond et al. 1989), but in practical terms it is only satisfactory to prescribe them for that purpose as part of a structured detoxification package.

### Prescribing benzodiazepines to methadone maintenance patients

This is a controversial area which arises frequently in the UK. Greenwood (1996) published results from the clinical treatment service in Edinburgh, in which impressive reductions in overall illicit drug use and drug injecting had been achieved with a prescribing policy which included benzodiazepines alongside methadone in two-thirds of cases. In the earlier influential studies which provided such strong support for the original model of methadone maintenance there was no benzodiazepine prescribing but, as we observed in Chapter 1, these often excluded individuals with polydrug use. Multiple drug use is now often the norm in those presenting for methadone treatment, and strategies to address substantial degrees of benzodiazepine misuse are increasingly required. There are no controlled studies of additional benzodiazepine prescribing to guide us, and so for the present the subject must be approached from a clinical perspective. In Table 2.3 I have attempted an analysis of the pros and cons of prescribing benzodiazepines in any more than the short term to drug misusers, the usual clinical situation in which this arises being ongoing methadone treatment.

One indication for prescription of benzodiazepines may be in individuals who are considered simply too dependent to withdraw successfully, just as is the case with a minority of ordinary-dose users. In such cases it is extremely important to restrict benzodiazepine consumption to the clinic's own supplies, and indeed one reason why a clinic may undertake some benzodiazepine prescribing is to be able to seal off other sources of supply, for instance from general practitioners. Different models of medical provision across countries mean that this is easier to achieve in some areas than others, and in general there is probably more sympathy for clinic benzodiazepine prescribing in systems where stopping other prescribing is relatively straightforward. Critics can point to the fallibility of such arrangements, the availability of benzodiazepines in the street drug scene, and the particular limitations of urine drug screening in separately identifying the different benzodiazepines.

More fundamentally in terms of clinical progress, some methadone patients appear to be able to stop using street drugs, notably heroin, if their prescription is augmented by benzodiazepines, when they have not previously been able to stop on methadone alone. It is possible to contend

Table 2.3. *Rationales for and against prescribing long-term benzodiazepines to drug misusers*

| For | Against |
| --- | --- |
| Some users too dependent to stop Control existing benzodiazepine usage | Promotes dependence |
| | Risk of erratic or dangerous usage |
| May help avoidance of street drugs | Benzodiazepine use associated with worse outcomes in some studies |
| Effective symptomatic treatment in individuals with poor coping resources | Prescribing can set unsatisfactory precedent |

that in such circumstances patients have been on inadequate doses of methadone, but clinically this does not always seem a sufficient explanation. The so-called 'opiate-enhancing' property of benzodiazepines probably produces a different effect to that of simply more methadone (Preston et al. 1984, Bell et al. 1990b), and while in services we generally do not wish to encourage drug combinations or 'dual dependency', taking the two drugs may be reasonably satisfactory in some cases. In many ways the issues for the prescriber are similar to those in stepping up to injectable methadone or an alternative more euphoriant opioid, always with the purpose of stopping street drug use; in this instance some individuals may have been taking heroin or cannabis to get to sleep, which benzodiazepines can replace. We also often encounter the situation of patients positively wishing to manage on a lower dose of methadone and, as discussed previously, we will not always stand in the way of this, even given the disadvantage of adding benzodiazepines. Finally, in terms of possible grounds for prescribing, the efficacy of benzodiazepines in treating anxiety and insomnia is readily appreciated by individuals who are not 'psychologically-minded', and have poor coping resources, and some clinicians may accept such a situation if they can take steps to see that misuse is not occurring.

Against prescribing, it seems inherently unsatisfactory in a drug dependence clinic to prescribe benzodiazepines with a regularity which may induce dependence, especially if this is not directly a response to previous benzodiazepine misuse. However, philosophically this is something of a dilemma: dependence (rather than adverse effects) has been identified as the main problem for ordinary dose licit benzodiazepine users but, in comparison with that group, if a drug misuser is already dependent on 80 mg of methadone per day is it more, or less, of an issue that they may become dependent on benzodiazepines? More practically, the risk of erratic usage is ever-present, particularly where the prescription systems which enable daily dispensing of methadone cannot stipulate this for benzodiazepines. The over-use of larger supplies has to be continually guarded against, with the worst consequence being fatality from combined drug misuse. As discussed in Chapter 7, studies of individuals who have died taking methadone show benzodiazepines and other sedatives such as alcohol to be frequently implicated (Worm et al. 1993, Risser & Schneider 1994, Clark et al. 1995) and, although the majority of such deaths involve outright abuse of methadone, the addition of benzodiazepines to a prescribed regime clearly increases the overall risk. The principles of making treatment as secure as possible, and the factors which have to be balanced against universal security, are discussed in detail in Chapter 7.

A series of studies in Sydney (Darke et al. 1992b, 1993, 1994a) found that benzodiazepine use in illicit drug users was associated with various adverse features, including poor physical and psychological health, more injecting, HIV-risk behaviours and polydrug use, and worse social impairment, although these were not studies of individuals prescribed benzodiazepines as part of a methadone programme. It should be noted that a very similar list of correlates is found in drug misusers who have personality disorder (Darke et al. 1994b, Seivewright & Daly 1997) – it may well be that the two aspects are related, or generally that benzodiazepine use tends to be an indicator of the more problematic cases of drug misuse. An important practical point in weighing the benefits and risks of issuing benzodiazepines to methadone patients is that any prescribing sets a precedent, in which benzodiazepines may be dubiously claimed as an entitlement when a patient presents elsewhere. As indicated above, this also applies in other prescribing situations, and such claims can be extremely troublesome in clinical practice. In our clinics we have taken the decision to issue no further prescriptions for temazepam to newly-presenting patients, partly because of the unfortunate precedent which prescribing sets – even though it might be justified in some individual cases. It can be argued that the particular problems resulting from injected abuse of temazepam (see Chapter 4) are less likely now that the capsules with liquid contents are unavailable, but the drug is still unduly sought after by illicit drug users and injection undoubtedly still occurs, and we feel that the benefits of avoiding such prescribing outweigh any limitations. It is made clear to patients that there are simply no exceptions to this rule, and we have had no significant problems in implementing the policy.

If a methadone maintenance patient does receive benzodiazepines, the implications for their treatment contract should be as if they had inject-able methadone or a more euphoriant opioid, although arguably the expectations may not be quite as high. The basic approach should be that since they have been given an additional medication with inherent disadvantages, probably because of an inability to stabilize on methadone alone, they must show abstinence from street drugs, otherwise there is no point in giving the additional medication. In some UK clinics benzo-diazepine prescribing is so widespread that this would unfortunately be seen as a counsel of perfection. The most justifiable reason for continuing a prescription of oral methadone plus benzodiazepines in the face of some ongoing drug misuse is if it effectively avoids the need for a higher level prescription, in somebody who would otherwise be a candidate. The most common such situation is where a persistent desire to use drugs by injection is reduced by benzodiazepines, enough to render an injectable prescription unnecessary, but not enough to result in complete cessation.

Finally, it should be stressed that not all benzodiazepine prescribing to methadone maintenance patients need be long term. McDuff et al. (1993) reported on detoxification from alprazolam, the benzodiazepine most commonly used by their methadone subjects. With methadone dosage usually remaining the same, patients were offered a set reducing course of alprazolam over 11 weeks. Of 22 patients, four refused the treatment and 12 out of 18 subsequently completed detoxification, although timescales in practice proved variable.

### Case history

Yousef is 27 years old and has been in methadone treatment for five years. He had previously used heroin for nearly as long, and initially in methadone treat-ment had found it very difficult to give up use of this drug. He would have heroin about once a week, with many urine samples positive and sanctions imposed at various stages. His other drug of preference was alcohol, and he would some-times attend the clinic intoxicated. There were generally limited expectations of progress, and he had few other social opportunities, being unemployed with no major qualifications. He had served one prison sentence and was regularly charged for being drunk and disorderly. He has always been very unenthusiastic about an increase in methadone, claiming to be quite comfortable on his 40 mg per day and to have other reasons for his heroin and alcohol use. He would drink in the daytime, not to alleviate withdrawal symptoms but more as a form of tranquillization, and about two years ago it was agreed that he could have some benzodiazepines prescribed to try and reduce his other drug use. It was made very clear that these would be stopped very quickly if there was no such improvement, and he was seen frequently during the early stages of benzo-diazepine prescribing. After various adjustments his prescription stabilized at methadone 40 mg per day, diazepam 25 mg per day and nitrazepam 10 mg nocte.

Although this approach is theoretically unsatisfactory, Yousef has proved able to avoid other drug use on the combination of methadone and moderate doses of benzodiazepines. He is never now intoxicated in clinic, and we have independent information that his drinking has greatly reduced. Most notably, all his monthly urine samples for well over a year have shown only methadone and benzodiazepines. He is regularly reminded that we are only prepared to give him benzodiazepines if we can see such clear progress, but he is adamant that this combination enables him to stop using other drugs.

### Alternatives to benzodiazepines

In any of the clinical situations in drug misuse where a benzodiazepine may be used, the less addictive alternatives should be considered. These fall into two groups: medications which are known from established usage to have very little misuse potential other than in exceptional individuals, and the newer alternatives to benzodiazepines, about which we can be less certain. In the first category, low doses of sedative antipsychotic drugs are commonly used for agitation in stimulant users, particularly in inpatients, and in some settings they feature in opiate withdrawal regimes. They may be tried as management of anxiety or insomnia, provided doses are well below the threshold of neurological side-effects, or some clinicians will use low doses of the sedative antidepressants, such as dothiepin, for sleeping problems. Trazodone provides sedation with the lowest level of antidepressant side-effects, while the least toxic option for night sedation is the antihistamine, promethazine. The second category of medication includes buspirone for anxiety, and zopiclone and zolpidem for insomnia, all of which produce less physical dependence than the benzodiazepines but are unlikely to be completely free of related problems. Zopiclone in particular has been associated with daytime misuse (Lader 1997), and is perhaps the most similar to the benzodiazepines in overall effects.

Although there are sound theoretical reasons for selecting these alternative medications, there is an ever-present problem of generally low acceptability in drug misusers. Unfortunately this is inevitable to some extent, given the links between acceptability and misuse liability for this population. Nearly all drug misuse clinicians would agree that benzodiazepine prescribing should be kept as low as possible, but such benefits as there are in a minority of cases probably depend on the particular agonist and subjective effects of those drugs. Also, as in low dose users, the alternatives are ineffective where there are withdrawal symptoms in cases of established benzodiazepine dependence, and the main role for these medications in drug misusers would appear to be in attempts to avoid initial exposure to benzodiazepines.

## Summary

The question of alternatives to methadone in substitution treatment in opiate dependence arises for various reasons. At the severe end of the caseload, there are many individuals for whom methadone does not enable good clinical progress, while for less dependent users there are emerging medications which, at least in theory, offer significant advantages.

One group of patients who are highly problematic in practice are those individuals who persistently use other drugs in addition to their prescribed methadone. In the original formal methadone programmes such patients were discharged, but now that there is more emphasis on retention in treatment this phenomenon is being witnessed increasingly. Critics of modern treatment claim that there are not enough additional elements in programmes to enhance motivation, or that methadone dosages are usually too low, but this is unlikely to be the whole story. Many patients cannot fully adjust to the noneuphoriant property of methadone, and either continue to use heroin in order to experience its particular effects, or attempt to enhance the effect of methadone by direct combination with other drugs. Some clinicians advocate the prescribing of diamorphine in such circumstances, with the added harm-reduction rationale that smokable diamorphine may be sufficient in individuals who are otherwise injecting drug cocktails.

The systematic evidence favouring diamorphine in some difficult long-term cases is increasing, but so far bioavailability problems of the smokable preparation have not been overcome. It would seem that diamorphine should at present be reserved for committed long-term injectors for whom other treatments have been unsuccessful, and such individuals are more likely to be engaged in treatment if this is offered, rather than for instance injectable methadone. Other euphoriant opioids may possibly be indicated in substitution treatment in particular circumstances, but there is virtually no supporting evidence from studies.

Methadone also has its disadvantages in patients who are less dependent and problematic. There is much concern about the drug's addictiveness and potential for fatal overdose, and buprenorphine offers advantages in these two areas and others. The claimed benefits of this drug, which also include less interaction with euphoriant drugs and quicker transfer to naltrexone maintenance, require further evaluation, with the combination preparation of buprenorphine and naloxone an interesting prospect. This is aimed at deterring misuse of buprenorphine tablets by injection, which was previously very problematic in street usage in the UK. At present dihydrocodeine is quite widely prescribed in cases of moderate opiate dependence, but this situation can easily degenerate and the drug is only really useful in set detoxification protocols.

The alternative agent which is most similar to methadone is levo-alpha-acetylmethadol (LAAM), with the important exception that it has a duration of action of up to 72 hours. This property is due to active metabolites, and is very advantageous in clinics which otherwise require methadone consumption to be supervised on a daily basis. With the UK treatment situation generally moving towards daily and on-site dispensing, LAAM could prove suitable for those patients who are progressing satisfactorily on methadone but for whom daily attendance would be unacceptable. Good motivation will be required to accept the use of a drug with slow onset of action and such periodic consumption, although this is only an extension of the principle of methadone treatment. LAAM will be indicated for similar patients to those who find methadone acceptable, rather than for the highly problematic group who may require a more euphoriant drug.

In the UK there has been some development of substitute amphetamine prescribing for dependent high-dose injectors of this drug. This is particularly controversial, and the number of services experimenting with some prescribing on pragmatic harm-reduction grounds is remarkable, given that national treatment guidelines have strongly discouraged this approach. Even the keenest proponents of amphetamine prescribing would concede that it is inherently much more unsatisfactory than prescribing for opiate users, but it would seem necessary for it to at least feature on the research agenda. At present there is something of a stand-off between opinion leaders who consider it simply unsuitable, and clinicians who observe that it produces benefits in some selected cases.

Prescribing benzodiazepines to illicit drug users is rather different in purpose, as use of these drugs is typically a subsidiary form of drug misuse. Severe benzodiazepine withdrawal symptoms may occur in polydrug users, and detoxification prescribing may be necessary in that context. Short-term benzodiazepine prescribing is also useful in opiate detoxification protocols such as those using lofexidine, but use in other circumstances is often risky, and sets a precedent which can be exploited by patients. The combination of benzodiazepines and methadone is extremely common, in a way that probably cannot be explained simply by inadequate methadone dosing. Relatively unproblematic low-dose benzodiazepine use must be distinguished from hazardous high-dose misuse, and some prescribing may be justified in association with methadone if this enhances control over supplies or eliminates use of street drugs.

# 3

## Achieving detoxification and abstinence

### Introduction

Whatever else a drug misuse treatment service does, it must be able to withdraw individuals from addictive drugs successfully. In recent years there has been much emphasis on methadone maintenance, partly on harm-reduction grounds, but meanwhile in the UK heroin has become readily available in most localities, and many users with short histories are presenting as suitable for detoxification treatments. In particular, young people are commonly turning to heroin after recreational use of amphetamine, ecstasy, LSD or cannabis, and are then often distressed by the development of physical dependence, which is in contrast to their previous drug experiences. A proportion of this group become committed heroin users, but many present for help to come off the drug, and typically do not want methadone or any other substitution treatment. Some drug services have found it difficult to adjust to this group of users, who may be reluctant to attend a place which they see as dominated by maintenance candidates, and who have very different treatment needs. In our services we consider the detoxification of young heroin users to be one of the main priorities in providing an effective community treatment response, and particularly in North Nottinghamshire we have gained much experience in this type of work. The first part of this chapter describes the methods we use for nonopioid community detoxifications, where we find that successful detoxification can be achieved almost as a matter of routine, *provided* that much attention is paid to both patient selection and to organization in treatment.

Individuals who are more heavily dependent on opiates clearly also require detoxification at various stages, and the remainder of the chapter discusses other forms of withdrawal treatment. As indicated in Chapter 1, community detoxification with methadone, as opposed to maintenance, is not well supported by evidence, but nevertheless this has been a standard treatment in the UK and other countries for many years. The place for methadone in withdrawal treatment will be discussed, as will the particular problems and practical aspects which apply to its use, and

Table 3.1. *Features desirable for quick community detoxification from heroin*

| |
|---|
| Short history |
| Low level of use |
| Not injecting |
| No significant current other drug use |
| Good motivation |
| Absence of personality disorder |
| Supportive family member(s) or partner to be involved |

the situation of pregnancy in which methadone needs to be the usual treatment. The last section discusses relapse prevention, focusing on counselling approaches and on the use of the opiate antagonist naltrexone, which we recommend after most detoxifications from opiates.

## Quick detoxifications from heroin

### Assessment, preparation and level of support required

Quick detoxification is a concentrated treatment approach, which requires motivation and organization on the part of both the drug user and the drug team worker. It is important not to attempt the treatment in unsuitable cases, and selection must be based not simply on whether an individual is 'saying the right things', but on relatively objective aspects of their drug use and situation which can predict outcome. Our experience points to the features in Table 3.1 as indicating likely successful completion of quick detoxification treatment.

A short history of heroin use is definitely desirable, preferably not more than a year to 18 months. The level of usage should be reduced during preparation for detoxification, but ideally has not been more than a gram per day (locally approximately 20% pure) at its peak. Current injecting usually counts against this form of treatment, and such users may be offered an intervening period on methadone so that they can give up injecting before having to give up opiate use; however, the population we see tend not to want methadone, and some users can convert from injecting to smoking once supportive counselling is underway. Significant use of any other drug makes uncomplicated completion of quick detoxification from heroin unlikely, while heavy previous usage, for instance a history of daily injected use of amphetamine, may also be a poor prognostic sign. Crucially, individuals must be well-motivated, and free from significant personality disorder, which appears to exert a generally adverse effect in detoxification attempts (Seivewright & Daly 1997). Finally, it is highly preferable if there is a family member or drug-free partner in the household to be actively involved in the detoxification, in terms of helping to manage medication and reducing the possibility of drugs being obtained at times of problems. Sometimes a couple will do this form of detoxification together, but it is unlikely to work if one partner or anyone else in the household is still actively using.

We find that a brief stage of preparation for the detoxification pays dividends, and no medication is issued at the assessment appointment. A urine sample is taken for drug screening to confirm the history, and the user is advised in standard drug counselling terms regarding taking responsibility for their own drug use and monitoring it, methods of cutting down, dealing with triggers and high-risk situations, and the assertive tactics in relation to lifestyle and drug-using acquaintances which will be necessary in retracting from the drug scene. At one or more further closely-spaced appointments the worker assesses progress, and detoxification starts when usage has reduced sufficiently, preferably to under a quarter of a gram per day.

Information on the withdrawal process is provided, along with schedules for the detoxification medications, and the treatment is also explained to anyone else who will be involved. Importantly, the detoxification takes place when the worker can fit in home visits through the period, preferably every day, and so it is not usually suitable to start a detoxification at a weekend. Given a well-organized service with competent drug workers, the only time a doctor need see the user is just prior to detoxification, to confirm that the method selected is suitable and to issue the prescription; the next involvement is to initiate naltrexone if detoxification has been successfully completed. This limited medical input can either be provided from the clinic, or by a user's general practitioner in liaison with the drug worker.

**Method 1 – Symptomatic medication**
Individuals on very small amounts of heroin are prescribed diazepam for anxiety, agitation or craving, nitrazepam for insomnia, hyoscine butylbromide (Buscopan) for stomach cramps, and diphenoxylate (Lomotil) for diarrhoea, over a seven-day period. The medication schedule provided to the user explains which drug is for which symptoms, and the maximum doses of each which can be taken in a day, which for diazepam varies during the course. The basic medication regime is included in Appendix 1.

## Method 2 – Lofexidine plus symptomatic medication

This is our main method of quick detoxification from heroin, suitable for most individuals of the type described in the assessment section above. The symptomatic medication options remain the same, but the principal treatment is lofexidine, an analogue of clonidine which does not have that drug's hypotensive effect and is therefore entirely suitable for community treatment. As a nonopioid method of controlling opiate withdrawal symptoms, it is an inherently appealing treatment to use in heroin users not severe enough to require methadone, and in the UK, one of the small number of countries in which lofexidine is so far available, it has been widely taken up by drug services for that indication. The drug is also useful as an alternative treatment at the end of a methadone detoxification, and in inpatient treatment and settings where methadone may be considered unsuitable, and these situations are discussed below. The claims for effectiveness have, until recently, largely been based on the similarity with clonidine (see below), plus early studies by Gold et al. (1981) and Washton et al. (1983), but support for lofexidine has now come from controlled studies (Bearn et al. 1996, Khan et al. 1997, Lin et al. 1997).

In our protocol the lofexidine dosage increases and then gradually decreases over six days, being at its highest when heroin withdrawal symptoms would be expected to peak. The medication regime is indicated in Appendix 1. The initial increase in dose is at a quicker rate than that recommended in the lofexidine (Britlofex) prescribing data sheet (Britannia Pharmaceuticals), but we find this most effective, and the prescribing information may be revised in due course as other services have apparently had similar experiences. In an inpatient comparison with methadone, Bearn et al. (1996) used the standard incremental increases in lofexidine up to ten 0.2 mg tablets per day, but considered that dosing to be probably suboptimal. In the standard regime, increasing to the maximum 12 tablets per day takes at least six days, but we prefer to make this available by the third day of a community detoxification, and find few problems when it is used. While the studies show little or no reduction in blood pressure, occasionally suggestive symptoms such as faintness on standing up are encountered, with low body weight females possibly particularly susceptible. Blood pressure should be checked before treatment and can be retested at visits, or for self-monitoring we instruct patients to check their pulse before a lofexidine dose, and to omit that dose if it is below 60 beats per minute.

**Case history**

Lee is 19 and works for a sports equipment firm. From the age of 16 he had used cannabis, LSD, amphetamines and ecstasy, but he claimed that none of this use had been heavy. He would use amphetamine, orally, about once every two weeks, and he liked to have one ecstasy tablet if he went to a nightclub. Ecstasy is the drug he would most want to continue, although he has been made aware of the risks. He has always kept himself fit, and sees recreational drug use as a normal thing for his generation.

His problem over the past year has been heroin, on which he became dependent following initial experimental use. After about three months he would get withdrawal symptoms if he did not have the drug daily, and his usage stabilized at 0.5 g per day, by smoking. He resented the control which heroin had gained over his life, and he could see that his general health was suffering. He told us 'I'm sick of heroin and I just want off it'.

Lee attended for a short series of counselling appointments to do the preparatory work for a detoxification. His parents had become aware of the problem, and after initial distress they were keen to help him through his treatment. With the counsellor's advice, Lee reduced his heroin use to the minimum which he needed to stop him withdrawing, and it was arranged that he had our standard detoxification regime of lofexidine and additional symptomatic medication. He had taken a week off work to do the detoxification, and daily home visits were undertaken.

Lee's progress through the detoxification was uneventful, with poor sleep the most troublesome aspect. He was pleasantly surprised with the low level of withdrawal discomfort, compared to his own attempts to come off heroin without medication. He and his parents followed the instructions carefully, and in all Lee used about three-quarters of the available medication, apart from the sleeping tablets which were all necessary. Nine days after his last use of heroin naltrexone was instituted, with no withdrawal reaction.

Three months later, Lee remains on naltrexone, and there has been no relapse into heroin use. He is enjoying sporting activities again, and has a holiday abroad planned with some friends. Although he had thought he would still use ecstasy, he appears not to have done so, wanting to try to manage without drugs altogether.

## Method 3 – Dihydrocodeine plus symptomatic medication

This is sometimes used for individuals whose heroin usage is not quite heavy enough to justify methadone, but who are considered unlikely to be able to tolerate a fully nonsubstitution method of detoxification. The drug is prescribed according to a fixed regime which is indicated in

Appendix 1, and which concludes with our usual combination of symptomatic medication. The course can be shortened, as suggested, if the relatively high doses in the first few days are considered unnecessary, or if it is felt there would be a problem in sustaining motivation over the 14-day period. Although this method has the disadvantage of delaying the introduction of naltrexone, because an opioid is used, it is useful for a service which emphasizes detoxification to make it available, for cases at a particular level of severity. We suspect that in future buprenorphine will prove suitable for this group, as discussed later in the chapter.

**Case history**

Jane is a 24-year-old single mother with two young children. Following occasional use of other drugs, she was introduced to heroin by her ex-boyfriend. He has had intermittent contact with drug services but proved to be poorly motivated, and he is now serving a prison sentence for supplying drugs. When Jane presented to our service recently she was smoking between 0.5 and 0.75 g of heroin per day, but wanted to stop all drug use and sever her contacts with the drug scene.

Jane had unsuccessfully attempted detoxification with lofexidine about six months previously. At the time she had been keen to have this method and then go on naltrexone, but the main problem had been that she was unable to reduce satisfactorily her heroin use in preparation. She also had the ongoing stresses of child care, although she had had some help offered.

Over the course of two counselling appointments it was clear that Jane would be unable to reduce her heroin substantially before a detoxification, but also that her general motivation was good. The dihydrocodeine method was selected, to give good symptom relief in the early stages of stopping moderate heroin usage. The nature of the treatment was carefully explained and the instructions were made very clear. A friend of Jane's had offered to have her children for much of the time during the detoxification period.

At three home visits during the first week it appeared that the detoxification was going according to plan. Jane felt comfortable on the dihydrocodeine until around the start of the second week, when she slightly overused the medication and the stage of symptomatic drugs had to be brought forward. With much support she saw the process through, and managed the nine days from the end of dihydrocodeine which we required before starting naltrexone. In the early stages following detoxification she has experienced some mood disturbance, and she is to be assessed for antidepressant medication.

## Clonidine

Clonidine reduces opiate withdrawal symptoms because it acts on the noradrenergic system, and some opiate withdrawal symptoms are due to noradrenergic overactivity. Specifically, it is an alpha-adrenergic agonist which acts preferentially on presynaptic alpha-2 neurones to inhibit noradrenergic transmission, with the action in the locus coeruleus particularly important in relation to opiate use (Gold 1993). The opiate withdrawal symptoms which have a noradrenergic basis include watery eyes, runny nose, sweating, diarrhoea, chills and gooseflesh, and so these are the ones usually relieved by clonidine and its analogues, lofexidine and guanfacine (Washton & Resnick 1981, Gossop 1988, Gold et al. 1981, San et al. 1990). Clonidine itself, however, has pronounced hypotensive and sedative effects which limit its acceptability and safety in drug misuse treatment. Although in inpatient detoxification with the drug some individuals may actually value the sedation and a related possible anti-anxiety effect, it is usually considered unsuitable for community treatment, when a less toxic analogue can be used.

## Methadone

Although in some countries methadone is considered as only suitable for maintenance treatment, in the UK it has also been the mainstay treatment for opiate detoxification. For very short-term detoxification its role is currently being reassessed in the light of the introduction of lofexidine and the presentation of many young, early-stage, heroin users who do not require or want substitution treatment, but clinics typically also have many individuals on slowly reducing methadone courses. Methadone in general and the role of maintenance treatment were discussed in Chapter 1, while this section examines the subject of detoxification with the drug in some detail, as in services where it is used it is often the main source of problems of practical clinical management.

### Suitability as a detoxification medication

Methadone is a hugely useful treatment in drug misuse, including in attempts at withdrawal, but unfortunately its portrayal as a detoxification method usually gives no indication as to how rare uncomplicated completion of treatment actually is. Figure 3.1 is a modified version of the schematic representation of methadone detoxification contained in the Department of Health's Guidelines on Clinical Management of Drug

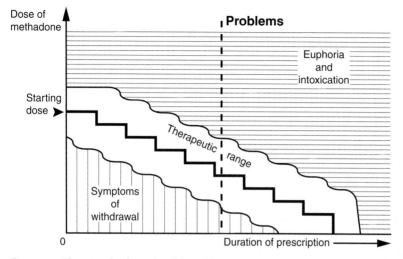

Figure 3.1. *The principle of opioid withdrawal by a reducing dose of methadone (adapted from Department of Health, 1991, reproduced with the permission of the Controller of Her Majesty's Stationery Office).*

Misuse and Dependence (1991) – the representation is the original, while the line indicating problems is my addition, reflecting previous observations such as those by Lowinson et al. (1976).

I would contend that in community treatment, the uncomplicated progress of a methadone detoxification by incremental reductions in dose from, say, 35 mg per day, 30, 25 . . . to . . . 10, 5, 4, 3, 2, 1, zero, establishing abstinence as planned at the end, is extremely rare, not to say virtually unknown. In practice many patients manage the first part, but requests will then be made not to reduce, or, if that is not an option, heroin use will re-emerge below a certain threshold dosage. In a medium-dose methadone detoxification, for instance starting at about 50 mg per day, problems will often be encountered at around 15 to 25 mg per day, the issue usually being severity of withdrawal symptoms, which even the best-motivated individuals will find it difficult not to seek to relieve in this relatively slow process. At such a stage decisions need to be taken as to whether to continue with methadone at a stable dosage for a period, whether even to increase to regain the benefits which have been lost, or to switch to one of the previously described methods of quick detoxification.

There seems little doubt that it is partly the properties of methadone itself, as well as factors relating to the users, which account for the difficulties seen in detoxification with the drug. The long duration of action and receptor binding properties which contribute to methadone's effectiveness as a stabilizing maintenance medication make it a much less suitable drug for detoxification, and presumably relate to the pervasive and protracted withdrawal symptoms which are frequently experienced. One of the most common observations about methadone is that 'it's worse to come off than heroin', and we should acknowledge that this is almost certainly true (Rosenbaum & Murphy 1984), to be weighed against the undoubted benefits of methadone in many situations. As well as seeing the difficulties of ongoing methadone detoxifications, many clinical workers operate with the assumption that withdrawal symptoms in any detoxification course will be worse if the detoxification is *from methadone*, than if the same course is used *from heroin*. Surprisingly few studies have directly tested this, but Gossop & Strang (1991) found that of heroin and methadone users given a ten-day methadone detoxification, the previous methadone users had more insomnia, muscular tension, weakness, and aches and pains, with completion rates similar in an inpatient setting, and dosage relatively unimportant. Certainly these symptoms are very familiar as generally the main complaints of individuals coming off methadone, with those who have done so in prison or residential rehabilitation often reporting that weeks or months have gone by before aching finally goes and sleep returns to normal.

In defence of methadone, the main difficulties some individuals have are of adjusting first to its noneuphoriant effect, and then to the prospect of being without drugs altogether (Milby et al. 1986). Methadone is used for more difficult candidates than nonopioid detoxification, and courses may become protracted partly due to actual reluctance to reduce, which compounds any difficulties relating to the drug. If detoxification has been imposed on an individual who is not ready to do it, the particular withdrawal syndrome of methadone is unlikely to be the critical factor, although it may not help.

A methadone detoxification is more often completed if it is done as an inpatient than as an outpatient (Gossop et al. 1986), but many individuals are reluctant to be admitted, and various other limitations of inpatient treatment were indicated in the Introduction. In attempting to provide the most useful combination of treatments in a community setting, we have no problem with offering methadone detoxification as an option, basically in cases where there are not the features favourable for the quicker methods. However, we do not expect it to proceed in a simple manner, and some of the more important practical management considerations are discussed below.

## Evidence from studies

Useful information on methadone detoxification as carried out in the UK has come from a series of studies at the Drug Dependence Unit of the Maudsley Hospital in London. In inpatient treatment, the prolonged opiate withdrawal symptoms in a methadone detoxification have been demonstrated, peaking towards the end of the course and lasting at least another 20 days (Gossop et al. 1987). Other inpatient studies have found that withdrawal distress is increased if individuals have high levels of anxiety (Phillips et al. 1986), and reduced if detailed information on the nature of withdrawal symptoms is provided (Green & Gossop 1988). A study which found similar levels of withdrawal symptoms in 10- and 21-day methadone courses (Gossop et al. 1989) led to the 10-day course being adopted as standard in that unit, but 10 days would almost always be considered too short for a community detoxification.

In a randomized controlled trial of inpatient and outpatient methadone detoxification (Gossop et al. 1986), completion rates were 81% in inpatients but only 17% (five individuals) in outpatients. Few details of the regimes are given, but the outpatient methadone course lasted eight weeks from an average starting dose of 37.5 mg, and abstinence was apparently confirmed by urinalysis. A study exclusively in outpatients investigated the matter of whether it was preferable to give users a say in their rate of detoxification, as opposed to imposing a fixed regime (Dawe et al. 1991). Users were randomly allocated to either a six-week methadone course which reduced at a set rate, or to a system where they could negotiate their rate of reduction, with the instruction that it was meant to last about the same period. Not surprisingly, only 17% (3) of the flexible group had completed their course by six weeks, the others having not reduced enough or dropped out. Approximately half of each group dropped out, and 40% of all urine samples during detoxification were positive for heroin – similar across the two groups.

## Practical issues

### Selection for treatment

Candidates for methadone detoxification can be seen as between those for quick detoxification treatments and those for outright methadone maintenance, in terms of severity of opiate dependence. Often, therefore, they would be 'beyond' the criteria referred to in the section on quick detoxification, with duration of heroin use more than 18 months, dose more than a gram per day, current injecting, other drug use, and/or adverse social situation. Some individuals' heroin use is not particularly heavy but for various reasons they find it difficult to reduce in preparation for a quick detoxification, and methadone may be more realistic in such circumstances. With others the social or home situation is the main problem, and the methadone option may be selected mainly in order to have a period on a stable dose to start with while other issues can be resolved. A user's previous experience with methadone or other detoxification methods also comes into the equation, but a fixation with methadone alone may be a sign of poor motivation for detoxification.

The consideration against outright maintenance treatment is only partly meaningful in the UK, as it is comparatively rare to accept at the start of methadone treatment that it will be definitely on a maintenance basis. This is a reflection of the dominance of slow outpatient detoxification as a model of treatment, which is discussed further below. In our own services we view a duration of dependent opiate use of about three years as something of a cut-off point, beyond which there should not be a strong expectation that detoxification can be achieved.

**Case history**

Martin is 28 years old and has been using heroin for two years, with little other drug use before that. His social scene has more usually involved alcohol, although Martin's drinking is not heavy. He works as a car mechanic, and is married with three children. His marriage has been under strain with his increasing heroin use, which has reached approximately 0.75 g per day. He has periods when he injects, but he has proved able to avoid this, especially when encouraged by contacts with the treatment service. Martin appears determined to overcome his drug problem, and is receptive to advice and counselling, and undemanding in terms of medication. He has never wanted methadone, and largely through his own choosing he has attempted detoxification four times, twice each with lofexidine and dihydrocodeine. He tries hard to see detoxification through, but he is drawn back to using heroin and he also has a tendency to over-use nitrazepam. For the first time he has recently started to become disillusioned about his prospects, and he has occasionally bought methadone from street supplies, which he says relieves his symptoms very well.

Martin is very opposed to the idea of receiving long-term methadone, which he sees simply as continuing dependence. We feel he now needs methadone, and we will provide a detoxification course. He is to start on 40 mg per day, with the plan to make reductions each four weeks. The most important aim in the early stages of treatment will be complete cessation of heroin and other drug use, to be monitored by weekly urine testing.

*Starting dose*

Methadone detoxification is nearly always in the form of the 1 mg in 1 ml mixture. Some individuals doing a detoxification from injectable maintenance wish to reduce in that form in the first instance, but clearly a switch to mixture should be made sooner or later, possibly using combinations of the two for a period. Methadone tablets are increasingly discouraged, while the 2 mg in 5 ml linctus may be useful at very low dosages, for ease of measurement.

Conversion tables from street heroin and pharmaceutical opioids are readily available (e.g. Preston 1996b), and one is included as Appendix 2. For a long time in the UK, rather conveniently, pounds in money of street heroin per day has approximately equated to requirement in mg of methadone, but the street values may well change. Such conversions of course follow assessment of reliability of information and confirmation of history, including urine testing. At one time admission to hospital for titration of dosage against withdrawal signs was fairly routine, but a titration approach is usually now considered impracticable in community treatment, if only because of numbers presenting. It is therefore necessary to be conservative in terms of the starting dosage, and this can be reviewed in the light of any remaining withdrawal effects at a subsequent appointment. It should be borne in mind that 70–75 mg of methadone would represent a lethal dose for an individual who proved not to be tolerant to opiates, and that death may occur at much lower doses than that if additional drugs are taken (Clark et al. 1995). For those who have had methadone unofficially in the street scene, it is useful to explain that the dose required in guaranteed daily treatment is less than they may have taken in an 'emergency' when withdrawing from heroin, in more erratic usage. Although formal titration has become less feasible, there are important issues to do with security of methadone treatment which are discussed in detail in Chapter 7. Because of the risk of overdose and fatality at the start of methadone treatment, it has recently been recommended that patients are informed of the risk and give written consent for methadone treatment, and that there should be frequent medical assessments in the early stages (Capelhorn 1998).

Individuals who have been misusing pharmaceutical opioids pose a particular problem, as any straight conversion from claimed average usage tends to result in methadone dosages which appear excessively high. In practice, such users can usually be given doses of methadone typical of routine treatment, as good progress is often made once the supportive elements of treatment are also in place.

Even in a short-term detoxification, an initial stabilizing period on the same methadone dose is often desirable, so that the user gains confidence in the treatment, and the effects of cessation of other drugs can be gauged before dose reduction. Further counselling on the withdrawal process can be done in this period, as typically some aspects do not 'sink in' while negotiation to secure methadone treatment is still underway.

*Dispensing intervals*
Although some users may be reluctant to agree to daily dispensing, it is difficult to argue a good case against it in the initial stages, when it is so important that the correct daily dosage is guaranteed. If it is unpopular, the matter of dispensing intervals can be used in a kind of behavioural approach, where there is some relaxation of the arrangement if good progress is shown. We prefer to revert to daily dispensing at the end of a detoxification, however, when small amounts are involved and stability is vital. Supervised consumption of methadone can readily be arranged not only at a treatment centre but also at community pharmacies (Scott 1996).

*Contracts*
The issue of contracts can be very unsatisfactory and causes much confusion in settings not geared to drug misuse treatment. Drug misusers as a group are prone to manipulation and will often seek to exploit any loopholes in agreements, and it is vital to be able to counter such situations confidently. Typically there is also resentment if 'new rules' are introduced part of the way through treatment, and the place for a clear unambiguous agreement about treatment conditions is at the start, in a maintenance or in a detoxification situation. In our services this is usually done verbally, with recording in the case notes, but occasionally a written contract is used, with each element signed, if there is cause to stress the contractual obligations particularly.

A treatment agreement or contract should cover required attendance at appointments, and the rules regarding abstinence from other drugs, and urine sampling. Some patients tend to comply with medical appointments but not counselling ones, and this may need to be addressed. It will normally be expected that urine samples become clear of other drugs soon after starting a methadone course, although there will inevitably be exceptional cases and circumstances, and some services pragmatically tolerate cannabis use, especially during a detoxification. Although it is easier to do the mandatory urine testing at clinic appointments, in our community service we have no problem in also making this part of the home visits from the drug worker, again having agreed this at the outset. One of our patients managed to provide a urine sample at his house which was temporarily without electricity and completely dark, with a torch held in his mouth to illuminate proceedings! Also specified in a contract are initial methadone dose, rate of reduction, any matters relating to additional medication, and the behaviours which will not be tolerated, such as abusiveness and aggression. Realistic sanctions are specified, including the step of premature reduction of methadone, and must be implemented if breaches occur.

If appointments are missed during a methadone course, the easiest way to regain contact is to withhold the next dispensing at the pharmacy until the patient has presented at the drug team. Given the nature of the treatment it is preferable for it to be reinstated within the same day, and so either the worker must be available or a temporary arrangement made where, for instance, a urine sample is obtained and the main appointment is rescheduled. For repeated non attendance the continuation of methadone, however, cannot be guaranteed, and for some contractual breaches the sanction will be termination of the methadone treatment, with a set period before another course can be provided. After any significant problem in treatment the nature of the contract should be reinforced at an appointment, and communication should be clear at all times, including with other professionals involved where sanctions have wider implications.

*Rate of reduction*
The practice of having an initial stabilizing period on the selected starting dose of methadone has been referred to, as has the strong likelihood of encountering problems with withdrawal symptoms towards the end of a detoxification. We expect to change to another form of detoxification when the methadone dose is down to about 10–20 mg per day, and we broadly acknowledge this with the patient, although attempting to avoid actually inducing problems through suggestion. Between these stages, there is simply not enough evidence relating to community (as opposed to inpatient) treatment to recommend any set period for a methadone detoxification, or therefore any particular rate of reduction. If it is unlikely anyway that a detoxification will be continued to its conclusion, the evidence of Dawe et al. (1991), referred to above, is not strong enough to definitely favour a fixed rather than a flexible schedule, and we offer users a say in the rate at which they will reduce. If the starting dose is, say,

40 mg per day, it might be proposed to reduce the daily dose by 5 mg each two weeks, or each four weeks, and it is useful to do the arithmetic with the patient and calculate how long a detoxification would take at that rate. The longer courses merge into the model of slow outpatient detoxification, which is discussed further below.

In quicker methadone detoxifications, some practical points can be important, such as having reductions take place between medical appointments rather than always being subject to discussion at the appointments themselves, when a user may be unduly tempted to delay the next move. Psychologically, some individuals who are motivated to detoxify nevertheless do not like to see their daily dose of methadone visibly reduce, claiming that this produces further anxiety, and for them we can provide a 'fixed volume reduction'. In this approach the volume of liquid remains the same while the methadone constituent gradually decreases, or to avoid excessive dilution at very low methadone dosages the volume may also reduce, but to a lesser extent. We adopt this method only when a patient has requested it, but by definition once the process is underway they are unaware of their exact methadone dosage, the pharmacist being requested not to divulge the information. In our experience this approach probably does not increase the rate of straightforward completion of methadone detoxification, but it can be effective in enabling substantial reductions in dosage in some cases.

*Additional medication*
It is preferable to use additional symptomatic medication only for specific opiate withdrawal symptoms, anxiety or insomnia when a switch is made from methadone reduction to another detoxification package (see below). The aspect of additional benzodiazepine use by methadone patients has been considered in Chapter 2, and can pose major practical problems in methadone detoxification. If benzodiazepines have been established alongside methadone maintenance treatment, then when the time comes for methadone detoxification there is often a temptation for individuals to at least want to continue the benzodiazepines, if not increase them to compensate for the reduction in methadone. Clearly, even if a methadone detoxification is successful there may then be an established high-dose benzodiazepine dependence to address, and the reality may be a confused situation somewhere in between. In short-term methadone detoxification, the temptation to add benzodiazepines for insomnia at an early stage should be resisted, as tolerance to the hypnotic effect of benzodiazepines occurs relatively quickly, and so by the time a user really

needs them, at the very end of a detoxification, they may have lost their effectiveness. Alternatives to benzodiazepines may sometimes be useful, as discussed in Chapter 2.

In addition to its use as a primary detoxification agent, lofexidine is used by some clinicians as an adjunctive treatment in a methadone detoxification, to help reduce the ongoing symptoms as reduction occurs. To us this does not seem the best way to use lofexidine, and a controlled study found guanfacine ineffective in this regard (San et al. 1994).

*Partial detoxifications*

If the difficulties encountered in a methadone detoxification are largely due to inability to tolerate the withdrawal features, the problems often start somewhere between one-half and three-quarters of the way through a planned reduction course. Problems much before this suggest other factors relating more to the individual, and in all cases when problems occur there must be a reappraisal of an individual's circumstances and of their prospects for detoxification. Sometimes it will appear that detoxification is too ambitious an aim, and that the individual may require long-term treatment. In other cases detoxification may still be desired, but an individual's personal or social situation may be conspiring against a successful outcome. Often a series of counselling sessions with a drug worker is required to make suitable plans, and the methadone dose may be held at the same level for a time-limited period while this is done. If a detoxification is to continue but definite problems with the reduction are being encountered, it is nearly always preferable to switch to one of the quick withdrawal methods outlined at the start of this chapter, if necessary with some modifications.

Although all three of the options can be considered, the option of symptomatic medication only is not usually sufficient for a detoxification from methadone (as opposed to low doses of heroin), while the relatively lengthy dihydrocodeine course arguably offers few advantages over a continued reduction using methadone. Sometimes, for individuals who have decidedly had enough of methadone a switch to a short dihydrocodeine course with the symptomatic medication can be suitable, but in this indication of partially-achieved methadone detoxifications the best option is the lofexidine course as previously described. We usually transfer completely from a low dose of methadone (preferably less than 20 mg per day) to lofexidine and the associated symptomatic medication, but some services use an overlap period of a few days in which methadone is reduced to zero while the lofexidine dose builds up. An account has been given of detoxification from methadone in the community using lofexidine, in which a group of established methadone users stopped the drug abruptly at an average dose of 35 mg per day five days into the lofexidine course, with satisfactory short-term completion (Eveleigh 1995).

It needs to be impressed upon patients who have been used to the comparatively lengthy timescale of methadone treatment, that the lofexidine detoxification package is time-limited – indeed, the reason for the change is to get the detoxification 'over with'. Because of the more pronounced difficulties in withdrawing from methadone as opposed to heroin, the prescribing of nitrazepam for insomnia may be slightly extended, but any tendency for benzodiazepines to become long term must be resisted, with alternatives investigated if necessary. The supportive elements of treatment are as important as when this form of detoxification is used from heroin, and sessions can be used to encourage abstinence from all medication.

### Slow outpatient detoxification

It would be difficult to overstate the predominance of this form of methadone prescribing in the UK. Patients start on doses of methadone which are adequate to relieve withdrawal symptoms comfortably and enable general well being, with a plan that the dose is gradually reduced over a period of months or even years. The context of this hybrid between detoxification and maintenance, which may be termed short-term maintenance, or 'maintenance to abstinence' (Department of Health 1991), has been discussed in Chapter 1. Reducing methadone rather than maintaining it outright may be seen as flying in the face of most of the evidence (Ward et al. 1998b), with reported rates of successful completion as low as 2% in a two-year reduction programme with strict conditions (McGlothlin & Anglin 1981). However, we have noted the marked selection issues in such research and the fundamentally changed nature of methadone treatment, and the clinical reality is that the majority of patients currently presenting to UK clinics with flexible prescribing policies have no wish to be on methadone indefinitely. It is certainly wrong to impose a withdrawal on severely dependent individuals, but many other patients are themselves concerned about the problems of long-term methadone, and wish to gradually reduce.

The whole range of rates of reduction is seen in clinics, from treatment that virtually constitutes maintenance, to shorter courses where the issues are mainly those which we have discussed above. At the more dependent end of the spectrum, there is little point in making small reductions so infrequently that a projected detoxification would take several years, especially if they have the result that the patient feels increasingly unwell, and risks losing the benefits of treatment. Such efforts tend to be poorly thought through, serving an unrealistic desire for eventual detoxification which may have come from either the doctor or the user. Advocates of maintenance treatment could undoubtedly point to a stable dose usually proving necessary in such cases, while it is inherently desirable for the aims of any treatment plan to be achievable.

A 'drift into maintenance' situation, in which a reducing course in a less dependent user goes on for substantially longer than originally planned, was noted in Chapter 1 to be partly the result of the various broader aims of methadone treatment, including harm reduction. For patients who become stuck halfway or so through a detoxification, we have observed that the best course of action is often to switch to an alternative treatment such as lofexidine. If, however, the user originally had more features indicating long-term treatment than very realistic prospects of detoxification, the outcome of ongoing low-dose methadone may in some cases pragmatically appear to be a reasonable one. This applies if the dose is sufficient to enable the user to feel well, to avoid other drug use, and make good general progress, but moderate enough to avoid intoxication or risk of diversion. In such circumstances there then needs to be a reappraisal with the patient of future prospects for detoxification and the overall objectives of treatment.

It is desirable for those undergoing slow methadone detoxification to also have drug counselling, from within the same treatment service. In a community-orientated service, most appointments can be with the non-medical worker, with the prescriptions provided automatically and medical input when required. If only the doctor is seen, the limited time tends to be mainly spent discussing medication reductions, with insufficient attention to other aspects. An assertive approach should be adopted in requiring attendance for counselling, and using those appointments to include realistic forward planning.

## Treatment in pregnancy

Prescribing for pregnant opiate misusers is considered here, as this usually takes the form of a detoxification with methadone. The particular situation of treatment in pregnancy has been reviewed by Jarvis & Schnoll (1994) and some important aspects are summarized in Table 3.2. Some

Table 3.2. *Treatment of pregnant opiate misusers*

*Presentation*
Often late
May be sensitive about statutory involvement

*Associated features*
Other risk factors for adverse foetal development
Partner often using drugs

*Liaison*
Antenatal and medical services
Social services

*Treatment*
Methadone where indicated, gradual detoxification if possible
Avoid benzodiazepines
Adjunctive symptomatic medication

opiate misusers realize only relatively late that they are pregnant, especially if they have amenorrhoea anyway due to the drugs. Other reasons may contribute to late presentation to services or to not volunteering a history of drug misuse, including fear of the reaction of authorities. In terms of clinical risk, there may be additional factors present which are associated with adverse foetal outcomes, including smoking, deficient diet and poor social conditions. These factors substantially confound the research on effects of the various drugs of misuse in pregnancy (Woods 1996), but heroin use and injecting are associated with prematurity, low birth weight and other obstetric problems which are reduced by methadone treatment (Wilson et al. 1981, Suffett & Brotman 1984, Jarvis & Schnoll 1994). The partners of pregnant users very often also use drugs, and it is important to attempt treatment with them also. If a partner does not commit himself to treatment and avoiding street drugs, this not only acts against the woman's chances of success, but may also put the future of the relationship under threat.

Compliance with antenatal care must be encouraged, and may be better if the antenatal and methadone services are linked. There should be testing for hepatitis B and C and HIV wherever possible, and liaison with the relevant medical specialties, as there are direct implications for vaccination or treatment of the babies. Testing is subject to widely varying policies and, while it is felt in the UK that HIV testing needs to remain voluntary at present, the current counselling-based approach is problematic in that it is associated with low uptake of testing antenatally (Gibb et al. 1998) and high rates of unrecognized vertical HIV transmission (Richardson & Sharland 1998). Liaison with social services is another very sensitive issue, but there are usually statutory guidelines for those working in drug services specifying circumstances in which child protection services must be alerted.

In terms of treatment for opiate misuse, a substantial proportion of women wish to detoxify during pregnancy so that the baby is not born addicted. It is very important that in generally accommodating this where suitable, there must also be consideration, in advance, of what the mother's treatment needs will be after delivery. A detoxification during pregnancy can be considered even less definitive than any other detoxification, as some women who will make a great effort to be drug-free at delivery may in other respects be likely candidates for long-term treatment. Treatment needs, including possible reinstatement of methadone if necessary, should therefore be assessed at all stages through pregnancy and after childbirth.

Even during pregnancy, detoxification should not be attempted in a long-term user if relapse to street drug use appears inevitable, or if it significantly occurs once detoxification is underway. Some such users will wish to reduce to the lowest feasible amount of methadone, which can be advised since there is probably a broad correlation between maternal dose of methadone at time of delivery and the occurrence of neonatal withdrawal symptoms (Maas et al. 1990, Doberczak et al. 1993, Malpas et al. 1995). Although we favour methadone reduction on these grounds, the issue is not entirely straightforward, as some studies fail to show a methadone dose – withdrawal symptoms correlation (Kaltenbach & Finnegan 1987, Mack et al. 1991), while a benefit of fewer neonatal withdrawal features may also need to be balanced against possibly less good foetal growth at lower methadone dosages (Hagopian et al. 1996). Many users who present, however, are quite capable of a full detoxification from opiates during pregnancy, particularly in this era of wider outreach and contact with many early-stage heroin users. Provided there is established dependence, methadone currently needs to be used for this rather than the quicker detoxification methods, as abrupt withdrawal should be avoided. In future, buprenorphine may also prove suitable for detoxification or maintenance treatment in pregnancy (Reisinger 1997).

Because opiate withdrawal stimulates uterine motility, it is conventionally advised to undertake detoxification in the middle trimester, with less risk therefore of miscarriage or premature labour. In practical terms, however, the time of detoxification depends substantially on the estimated risk of return to street drug use between the end of detoxification and delivery, and also on when the user presents and her level of usage. The calculations in a planned methadone reduction course are based on these factors and on the principle of reducing sufficiently slowly, probably by not more than 5 mg in the daily dose each two weeks. In this way a methadone withdrawal regime may often continue into the late stages of pregnancy, especially when presentation for treatment has been delayed. Benzodiazepines should preferably be avoided in early pregnancy as they may be associated with foetal malformations (Dolovich et al. 1998), but symptomatic relief may be aided by antispasmodics for stomach cramps.

### Case history

Julie was 20 years old and pregnant for the first time. She presented to our service at the early stage of eight weeks of pregnancy, encouraged by her boyfriend who was a patient of ours. He was on moderate-dose methadone, but was known to additionally use heroin quite regularly. It transpired that he did this with Julie, who had a heroin habit of about 0.5 g per day. She had used the drug for about a year, having injected on only a very few occasions.

Since finding out that she was pregnant, Julie was very keen to detoxify from heroin. Her initial reaction had been to stop quickly by herself, but she had been advised that this could be dangerous. It was explained that she would need methadone treatment, but she wanted to be off all opiates by the time of delivery, and her boyfriend indicated that he would reduce and come off methadone at the same time. A detoxification had not otherwise been planned for him, but he had decided he was 'fed up with it all anyway' and they did not want to be using drugs as parents.

Julie was nervous about going to antenatal clinic, and she was helped with arrangements to attend the service which specializes in seeing drug users, among other groups. She had hepatitis and HIV testing at the genito-urinary medicine department and was found to be negative for both conditions. In the short period between assessment and starting methadone treatment she managed to reduce her heroin use slightly, and 30 mg of methadone per day was enough to alleviate withdrawal symptoms comfortably. Her daily dosage reduced by 5 mg each three weeks down to 15 mg per day, with two reductions then to 10 mg per day, and weekly reductions by 1 mg in the daily dose thereafter.

She was known to use heroin on three occasions during the detoxification, with several other clean urine samples. Her boyfriend did not manage his detoxification, but on reestablishing ongoing treatment he undertook to use no heroin or other street drugs. He used heroin on the same occasions as Julie, with again other evidence that he was successfully avoiding the drug. Although there were no complications of pregnancy, Julie was admitted to the antenatal ward at her own request for two weeks prior to delivery, to ensure that she would be using no drugs. Delivery was uncomplicated, and her baby boy showed no signs of opiate withdrawal effects and was discharged home after a short stay. We consider that Julie is at significant risk of relapse into heroin use, and are continuing to see her, along with her boyfriend.

## Buprenorphine

In Chapter 2 we identified that buprenorphine may have four possible advantages over methadone for use in clinical treatment. Buprenorphine appears to be safer and less addictive, while there are also fewer interactions with other euphoriant drugs, and a shorter time interval necessary between its use and starting naltrexone treatment. The second and fourth of these are particularly relevant to the use of buprenorphine as a detoxification treatment.

We have noted that the extent to which difficulties occur when a reducing course of an opioid substitution agent is used for detoxification relate both to any previous maintenance treatment with the drug, and to newly emerging symptoms in the withdrawal process itself. In contrast to methadone, the withdrawal from chronic buprenorphine treatment has been shown in animal and human studies to produce a mild abstinence syndrome, even when withdrawal is precipitated by opiate antagonists (Negus & Woods 1995). It will probably, therefore, prove easier to detoxify from buprenorphine than from methadone after long-term treatment, while buprenorphine itself may be a suitable detoxification agent in withdrawal from heroin. In an early study (Bickel et al. 1988) buprenorphine was found to be as effective as methadone in this regard, with an intervening stabilizing period on 2 mg per day and 30 mg per day, respectively, while symptom relief in short-term detoxification from heroin has been found to be better using buprenorphine than clonidine (Cheskin et al. 1994).

Naltrexone treatment in its relapse prevention indication can be started virtually immediately following a buprenorphine detoxification (Rosen & Kosten 1995), as opposed to the delay of ten days which is necessary from the end of methadone treatment (see below). The combination of this advantage, less addictiveness than methadone, and apparently good symptom relief will make buprenorphine a very interesting candidate for opiate detoxification as it becomes generally available in the UK. We would see one likely target group as those heroin misusers who are too dependent to be suitable for detoxification with lofexidine, but who do not definitely require methadone, a group in whom we are currently using dihydrocodeine (see page 86).

The apparent advantages of buprenorphine raise the possibility of transferring individuals from methadone maintenance to this drug to facilitate easier withdrawal. This aspect has been investigated in inpatients (Walsh et al. 1995) and in one UK outpatient setting (Law et al. 1997).

## Inpatient treatment

The general issues concerning inpatient treatment of drug misusers have been discussed in the Introduction, and the use of methadone as a detoxification treatment earlier in this chapter. Many of the problems of methadone detoxification, including the risks of misuse and diversion, and noncompletion due to inability to tolerate the prolonged withdrawal effects, are reduced in inpatient treatment, and use of the drug remains a valid approach in that setting, with the various provisos referred to above. However, the methadone courses may last three weeks or even more, and with length of stay identified as an important issue by both patients and treatment providers, there is currently much interest in regimes which can achieve detoxification from opiates more quickly.

As indicated, buprenorphine may offer a quicker option than methadone, with a three-day course reported to be effective for withdrawal from heroin (Cheskin et al. 1994). The side-effects of clonidine which render it unsuitable for community treatment can be manageable in the inpatient setting, although the drug is being superseded by lofexidine where that is available. Recent controlled studies have found clonidine and lofexidine to be equally effective in alleviating withdrawal symptoms in inpatient detoxification from heroin (Lin et al. 1997) and from methadone (Khan et al. 1997), with lofexidine resulting in less hypotension and fewer adverse effects. Another double-blind controlled study found lofexidine to be broadly as effective as a ten-day methadone detoxification in inpatient opiate withdrawal (Bearn et al. 1996).

The terms rapid opiate detoxification, or accelerated withdrawal, are used to refer to techniques in which withdrawal is actually precipitated by administration of an opiate antagonist, and then nonopiate drugs are used to manage the symptoms. Various regimes have been described, using either naltrexone or intravenous naloxone at the outset, and clonidine, lofexidine and various sedatives (e.g. Bartter & Gooberman 1996, Merrill & Marshall 1997). The most severe techniques are carried out under heavy sedation or even general anaesthesia (Loimer et al. 1991a, Brewer 1997, Tretter et al. 1998). Rapid detoxification, particularly under anaesthesia, has received a good deal of publicity, and can catch the imagination of older users in particular who still retain a desire to detoxify, but have become disillusioned with conventional, longer methods. Increasingly, a distinction seems to be being drawn between the relatively well-tried methods virtually confined to naltrexone and clonidine or lofexidine, and the more severe experimental techniques. For instance, in a brief report, Rumball & Williams (1997) make claims for their routine method over eight years' experience, and consider that, by contrast, 'it is the introduction of anaesthesia and polypharmacy to the process that has … quite unnecessarily introduced major hazards'. They report high acceptability, provided patients are excluded who may also be withdrawing from benzodiazepines or alcohol, have used large or unquantifiable amounts of opiates, or have serious physical illness or lack of venous access. The basic rapid detoxification techniques have indeed become widespread, partly through a desire to make more efficient use of inpatient units. It should at least prove possible to reduce the proportion of individuals who fail to complete a detoxification, if only because the time period involved is shorter.

It is, however, detoxification under general anaesthesia which has attracted the most publicity in the media, and in my experience the most interest on the part of community patients. It is often alleged by drug misuse specialists that a condition which is not itself dangerous, opiate withdrawal, does not justify the risks of an anaesthetic. However, proponents of the method point out that the same argument is not always used in, say, childbirth or dental treatment, and there is a case for weighing the risks of anaesthetic against not only those of withdrawal, but also those of ongoing drug misuse. That case would be stronger if it were shown that detoxification under anaesthetic led to higher abstinence rates than other methods, but that so far remains unknown.

There is clearly further debate among those who carry out the different ultra-rapid experimental techniques as to whether the risks of an anaesthetic, in a relatively young person without any invasive procedure being performed, are actually greater than those where very high doses of oral sedatives are managed by a psychiatrist, but no useful comparisons are yet available.

## Other influences on choice of detoxification method

Ideally, the detoxification treatments selected for individuals should be the ones most suited to their drug history, taking into account the available evidence, and to some extent their own views. In all clinics the permutations have to be limited to some degree in order to provide equitable treatment, but in some other settings major treatment options may be excluded on policy grounds, typically methadone where there are reservations about prescribing controlled drugs. A common example is prison, where although it may be argued that methadone maintenance is especially indicated because of high rates of needle sharing and other HIV-risk behaviours, often treatment is limited to short-term symptomatic medication for initial opiate withdrawal symptoms. Another is the case of primary care practices which may wish to offer some treatment to drug misusers, but are not prepared to use controlled drugs.

In community treatment, it is important to be able to work with primary care physicians with varying prescribing policies, but we should not be drawn into giving inappropriate treatments. The reluctance of a doctor to prescribe methadone is not the right reason for a drug user to be given benzodiazepines or dihydrocodeine. A prison inmate with a substantial heroin dependence who is given short-term symptomatic treatment may simply suffer (depending on availability of drugs), but such an individual in the community will inevitably continue to use drugs, and views on the ineffectiveness of treatment can become reinforced. In practice, a community drug team should be involved in both liaison and training to encourage treatment in general practice, but should also ensure that the full range of treatments are available through its own clinic as a back-up, so that methadone, for instance, can be provided where necessary. In the UK, lofexidine is once again proving a useful mid-range treatment option in the prison setting and widely in general practice.

## Treatment of minor opioid misuse

Primary misuse of the minor opioids, such as dihydrocodeine, codeine or dextropropoxyphene (this usually in combination prescriptions) gets little recognition, but it can be very troublesome in clinical practice, and requires strategies for management. One reason why there is hardly any systematic literature is that this form of drug misuse rarely presents to specialist services, with general practitioners more likely to be alerted by escalating prescriptions. Our impression of dextropropoxyphene misuse in particular is that it is more common in women, typically with long-standing personal or psychological problems who may also use tranquillizers or alcohol, but other populations have been described (Ng & Alvear 1993).

If usage is heavy enough, pharmacological detoxification may be required, along with appropriate counselling. Lofexidine may be useful in the protocol described earlier, or in severe cases methadone may be required over varying time periods. Typically there is low acceptability of methadone, with users tending to make the case for their own drug of preference if there is to be ongoing prescribing, just as can occur in those who have become dependent on opioids for pain relief. Methadone is perceived as being for illicit drug abusers, and for those on prescribed minor opioids there are not the same social reasons to have to switch to that drug. Nevertheless, methadone should usually be used if detoxification needs to be gradual, with dosage based on standard conversion charts (Preston 1996b), also taking the drug half-lives into account. Where the drug of misuse has been a combination product of dextropropoxyphene and paracetamol, if methadone is to be avoided a reducing course of dextropropoxyphene only can be prescribed, thus avoiding liver damage from the paracetamol component.

## Relapse prevention

### Naltrexone
Naltrexone is a long-acting competitive opiate antagonist which is effective orally (Gonzalez & Brogden 1988). It can be used to precipitate withdrawal in accelerated detoxification from opiates (see above), but its main use in community treatment is as a relapse prevention strategy (Farren 1997). The principle of treatment is that on establishing a dosage of one 50 mg tablet per day, any ordinary amounts of opiates which are subsequently taken are rendered completely ineffective, the medication therefore acting as a strong disincentive to drug use. This resembles the use of disulfiram in alcohol abuse, but with the great advantage that there is no dangerous interaction to guard against, and so it can be used much more freely. In our regimes for quick detoxification from heroin which I have described above, naltrexone is an integral part of the treatment package, which users are briefed about from the start. Indeed, given the general difficulty of staying off heroin in communities where it is freely available, increasingly we find individuals presenting whose main

motivation is to have treatment with 'the blockers'. In turn, one of our reasons for selecting lofexidine as the main method of detoxification, or in the mildest cases symptomatic medication only, is that naltrexone can be established straight away on completion of the detoxification, since an opioid has not been used. This combination approach is often attempted in UK services, but we feel that to be successful with this type of user naltrexone must be assertively encouraged from the outset. Our view – and apparently that of the users – is that relapse rates in opiate misuse are such that there needs to be a good reason *not* to include this relatively straightforward treatment option, for a period, in attempting to enhance an individual's chances of success.

The effectiveness of naltrexone in this indication has been demonstrated in controlled studies (Shufman et al. 1994, Gerra et al. 1995). It is generally recognized that naltrexone treatment should be in the context of some form of counselling on avoiding relapse, while Brewer (1993) has stressed the importance of consumption of the medication being supervised, for instance by a family member. Probation-linked supervised naltrexone has been used as an alternative to custody in opiate-misusing offenders (Brahen & Brewer 1993). So long as there is a 50 mg dose for each day, treatment can be given three times or even twice per week, although if the supervision is at home the daily regime is perhaps easier to remember.

The tablets may be crushed up in a liquid, preferably something like a fruit juice as there is a bitter taste. No depot preparation is yet available for routine use. Naltrexone should probably not be used in those with significantly impaired liver function, as abnormal liver function tests have been demonstrated in treatment with a much higher dose, used for obesity. Side-effects at the 50 mg dose may include headaches, dizziness, nausea, and feelings which resemble mild withdrawal such as chills or abdominal discomfort. Various mood disturbances are common in the early stages of treatment, but these may often be related to the absence of mood-altering drugs and the general process of adjustment, producing for instance some frustration or irritability.

Because of the nature of naltrexone treatment it is clearly necessary to have been opiate-free for a period before starting. An interval of 7–10 days is usually recommended, the lower number if the withdrawal has been from heroin and the higher if from the longer-acting methadone. If a nonopioid method of detoxification is employed, the days in this treatment can of course be included if no opiate use has occurred. The manufacturers of naltrexone have recommended that a challenge with intravenous naloxone is performed to detect, by the presence or absence of precipitated withdrawal symptoms, whether the period off opiates has been adequate. Increasingly, however, services are using a small dose of oral naltrexone itself for this purpose. In common with others (Brahen & Brewer 1993), we find that in detoxification from small amounts of heroin the opiate-free period does not need to be as long as seven days, and that naltrexone can often be introduced cautiously from about four days onwards. Our users are often impatient to start, and indeed derive a strong psychological advantage from doing so, and treatment can be initiated at a quarter of a tablet for a day or so, moving to half a tablet and then the full one tablet per day by the standard 7–10 day opiate-free stage. Supervision of the first dose by the worker is desirable, with 30–60 minutes' observation for withdrawal symptoms.

There is little evidence to bring to bear on the question of how long naltrexone treatment should continue. Several studies have used a six-month period, including one which found no advantage of naltrexone over placebo, notably in polydrug users with lengthy histories (San et al. 1991). As with disulfiram, there is probably no set period which is preferable, with much individual variation in availability of supervision, extent of exposure to risky situations, motivating factors, and toleration of the drug. We routinely use naltrexone for four weeks in the initial period of adjustment after detoxification, and then recommend continuation for three to six months if there are no problems of acceptability. It is not uncommon for users to test out naltrexone by having an amount of heroin, and, although any drug use in such circumstances is unfortunate, at least it is then recognized that the blockade does indeed work. 'Overriding' the effects of naltrexone probably requires taking four or five times an average heroin dose, and is not attempted in the population in which we are using the medication.

It is possible to have various reservations about naltrexone treatment, and there are clear limitations as well as some potential for what may be broadly termed misuse. Brewer (1996) has criticized the ideological objection to naltrexone, from those who believe that motivation to abstain from drugs can only truly come from an individual's personal psychological resources. Recognition of relapse rates is probably sufficient for most clinicians to avoid adhering to that position rigidly, but the view is encountered in some settings which practice particular purist treatment models, such as some residential rehabilitation centres. More in terms of general clinical impressions, some workers feel that naltrexone probably works best in those who would have managed well without it anyway, but this has not really been tested and is not in itself an objection to the treatment. A definite limitation of the treatment is that it clearly only acts in relation to opiates, and so cannot prevent relapse into other drug misuse.

In using naltrexone treatment widely, we have occasionally encountered various inappropriate usages of the medication. One type of situation extends out of the proper use, but without full compliance of the patient. Thus, a relative or partner may insist on naltrexone being continued even when they suspect that relapse has taken place, or alternatively they may resort to concealed administration. One woman who was exasperated by her partner's failure to take the medication put it in his cup of tea, but unfortunately their friend who was an active user drank this by mistake, and promptly became very ill with withdrawal symptoms. Some parents have realized that giving naltrexone can test whether their child is on heroin, and one teenager presented to us in severe withdrawal having had this done. Drink-'spiking' with naltrexone is also emerging, seemingly done to users by their friends for amusement purposes. Users themselves may misguidedly decide to take naltrexone to attempt a quick self-detoxification, which is a potentially dangerous situation, particularly in impulsive heavily dependent polydrug users. All these inappropriate uses have implications for the security of naltrexone treatment, which requires a good degree of reliability on the part of patients and their associates who will supervise the treatment, or otherwise controlled dispensing conditions. Our experience has mainly been with well motivated early-stage heroin users, very different from the forensic or professional groups with whom naltrexone has sometimes previously been associated, and in general we find very high levels of acceptability and a low rate of treatment-related problems.

A recent development in treatment has been to combine giving naltrexone with prescribing the serotonergic re-uptake inhibitor fluoxetine, in view of that drug's possible effect in reducing drug craving (Sellers et al. 1991) (see page 122). Following earlier case reports, a randomized controlled study from the Basque country in Spain has demonstrated improved retention rates when fluoxetine was added to naltrexone maintenance in a relapse prevention programme for heroin addicts (Landabaso et al. 1998). The authors suggest that placebo-controlled studies are required to test whether this is a specific effect while, in general, if fluoxetine or another antidepressant is beneficial this may be due to direct relief of depressive symptoms, which appear common in the early stages after detoxification.

**Case history**

Kerry had a one-year history of heroin use before undergoing a straightforward community detoxification with lofexidine and symptomatic medication. She was keen to go on naltrexone, and we supervised the first half-tablet dose, eight days after her last use of heroin. Her mother had helped her through the detoxification at home, and was also going to make sure that Kerry had her naltrexone each day. They were given a patient information leaflet, and a medical warning card for Kerry to carry with her at all times.

Taking naltrexone posed no problems, with her mother good at remembering and, particularly in the early stages, checking to see that Kerry had not secreted the tablet in her mouth. They had a good relationship and Kerry had no objection to the situation being managed in this way. She initially experienced some headaches, but after a week on the medication these went away.

Kerry was regularly seen by her drug worker during treatment with naltrexone. She checked whether she could use cannabis and alcohol while on the medication, and did continue to use these intermittently. On one occasion only, she 'tested out' the naltrexone by using heroin, but reported that she had no effect from the drug. She also said that she generally did not crave heroin, and clearly saw this as a consequence of being on naltrexone – 'because you know you can't have it, you don't wind yourself up thinking about it'.

After four months Kerry considered that she was at very little risk of using heroin again, and did not want to take the naltrexone any more. She felt that taking the tablet was itself an unnecessary reminder of heroin, which she would manage to avoid because she was determined not to go back to her previous lifestyle. Her mother was nervous about this change, but at subsequent monthly appointments, which Kerry had still requested, there has been no evidence of relapse.

## General methods

Not all those who have stopped taking opiates, or drugs in general, require counselling in relapse prevention. It has been observed that cigarette smokers who give up mainly get on with consolidating abstinence themselves, and do not have sessions discussing personal issues. Certainly it can be a mistake to bring recently detoxified drug users back to a busy clinic, where they will find the waiting-room conversations about drugs distressing, and there may be attempts by others to undermine their abstinence. However, we find that many users who have had contact and support through a community detoxification do want to continue seeing their worker for a period afterwards, when various difficulties may be encountered. We offer this in the form of home visits,

Table 3.3. *Areas to cover in relapse prevention counselling*

Tactics in avoiding active drug users
Dealing with craving and trigger situations
Making realistic short-term plans
Time management
Reinforce need for complete abstinence from drug

to ensure contact and also because group meetings can be too risky in the early stages. We favour relapse prevention groups for alcohol misusers, but with drugs there is probably a higher risk that one individual who has relapsed will 'bring the others down', for instance by bringing drugs in. Where an individual does request ongoing visits and counselling, we do this for as long as it appears useful at increasingly spaced appointments, often tied in with naltrexone treatment.

The principles of relapse prevention counselling are similar across the range of drugs, the main theoretical influences being the work of Marlatt & Gordon (1985) and the technique of motivational interviewing (Noonan & Moyers 1997). Drug workers of all disciplines carry out such counselling, and practical guides from the nursing perspective have been provided by Wanigaratne et al. (1990) and Salazar (1997).

A wide range of adjustments need to be made after detoxification, in many different individual circumstances. Long-term methadone maintenance patients who detoxify may have few or no peers who are nondrug users and little remaining from a drug-free lifestyle, with therefore much rebuilding to do. Younger heroin users who go through a quick detoxification, as described at the start of this chapter, usually have a more intact social situation but have to make their adjustments to being abstinent in a very short period. Overall, the practical issues which our team workers find most important to address after detoxification are indicated in Table 3.3.

Avoiding acquaintances who are still using drugs is usually crucial, however solitary it renders an individual's situation (hopefully temporarily). Other users may be envious and attempt to continue contact as if nothing had happened, and dealers do not take kindly to losing a regular customer. Families and partners can be involved in rejecting such approaches, and the worker can help advise on the tactics required. One of our clients wrote to us about the difficulties of separating from other users after detoxification:

You are probably aware that the heroin culture that is quickly emerging, is based on a sense of kinship, a need to belong to an identifiable group. While in this group, young people find that sense of belonging that is missing, whether due to unemployment, or other problems. Subsequently the descent into a habit they simply cannot afford to sustain by normal means is swift. The route out of the habit is not so easy, largely because of the fact that ex-users are subsequently shunned by their peers. I would go as far as to draw the analogy that going 'clean' is tantamount to one of a group of burglars suddenly joining the Police. This in turn regenerates the feeling of isolation that being a user suppresses, and so it is easier to stay on the stuff than to be subjected to the stigma of coming off.

Craving can be problematic, as can trigger situations, usually localities or having money. The day on which a benefit payment or wage is received is especially difficult if money has previously translated into drugs, and tactics are required to spend it on necessities or other things that are desired. Dealing with craving usually involves various methods of distraction, suitable for each individual. Planning new activities is important, but this must be realistic and involve definite action in the short term. Thus if going to college is planned, this involves obtaining information, making decisions about courses and submitting applications at organized times, with guidance. There is usually a vacuum of time to fill in the initial stages, in contrast to previous involvement in raising money and using drugs, and time management advice is useful. Also some 'myths' about drug use can require de-bunking, particularly where individuals feel they could safely use their drug occasionally on a 'treat' basis – the impossibility of doing this with heroin in particular often needs stressing.

Boredom is a great enemy in this situation, with great differences between areas and countries in the likelihood of gaining employment. In our areas unemployment generally is at high levels, and drug users can feel as if they have few or no prospects. There is no establishment of special schemes whereby users who have detoxified can secure employ-ment as part of rehabilitation, and we often have to provide much encouragement and practical help to seek the few opportunities that there are. The probation service can sometimes offer places on schemes for ex-offenders in particular.

The biggest single adjustment which has to be made on detoxification is that to being without the effects of a mood-altering drug. Clearly, some revert to heroin because of an inability to make this adjustment, but others will switch to a different drug, perhaps one they used earlier in their 'career', or commonly alcohol if they have determined to try to do without drugs. Alcohol is in some ways a particular risk, as those wishing to separate from the drug scene can aim to reintegrate with their previous friends who 'just go out drinking'. Where alcohol use does become excessive shortly after giving up opiates we often find this to be a phase which subsides, but there can come a point where alcohol or any other drug misuse becomes problematic enough to require treatment in its own right or, where relevant, to raise the possibility of reestablishing previous maintenance methadone. The study by Eklund et al. (1994) which illustrates this phenomenon in relation to detoxification from methadone was discussed on page 24.

**Special methods**

Clinical psychologists are not very numerous in community drug services in the UK and, as already noted, counselling techniques originally derived from this discipline are usually carried out by other workers. Something of a balance needs to be struck here: psychological methods are most purely administered by clinical psychologists, but counselling clearly needs to be more widely available, and drug users can be scathing of generic therapists who 'don't know anything about drugs', typically failing to comply if they perceive that to be the case. We would tend to look to input from clinical psychology, preferably within a drug service but if necessary from elsewhere, in cases where risk of relapse appears to be related to long-standing problems of a psychological nature. Some drug users appear to 'self-medicate' to relieve distress from painful previous experiences, of which child sexual abuse is prominent, and this phenomenon needs addressing if abstinence from drugs is attempted. Where family dynamics appear an important causal or perpetuating factor in an individual's drug misuse, systematic family therapy is another area which requires specialist handling.

Many drug misusers derive benefit from the Narcotics Anonymous organization, whose methods are well known and importantly include an unequivocal commitment to total abstinence from all substances, regular attendance at meetings, and a fellowship of ex-users who can be contacted for support (Cook 1988). Our own experience is that this approach finds favour with only a relatively small minority of the users who attend clinical services, noticeably smaller than the proportion of alcohol misusers who respond to the generally better-established Alcoholics Anonymous. Probably subcultural differences between the two groups are important, while also our young drug users typically cannot comprehend a future without social use of alcohol, risky though this is.

## Summary

The widespread availability of heroin in the UK means that very large numbers of users take this drug in effect as an extension of recreational drug use. A common pattern is that users of amphetamine and ecstasy in the nightclub drugs scene take heroin as broadly an alternative to cannabis, tranquillizers or alcohol to 'come down' from their stimulants, and in due course become dependent on the opiate. Many young users are presenting to services with the aim of a quick withdrawal from heroin, and this group have very different treatment needs from the longer-term opiate users, for whom the harm-reduction benefits of maintenance treatment are often emphasized. Although there is not yet substantial systematic evidence, clinical services are finding that the young users easily manage to detoxify, provided there is adequate attention to initial preparation and then support through treatment.

Lofexidine, a clonidine analogue without the hypotensive or sedative side-effects, is ideally suited to community detoxification of early-stage heroin users. Our preferred treatment package is a one-week course of lofexidine plus various symptomatic medications, while for very mild cases we will use only the symptomatic medications, or for more severe cases a set dihydrocodeine detoxification. Patients have daily home visits through the withdrawal period, and there is high acceptability of this management approach. Our guidance at present is that quick detoxification using lofexidine is most successful where there is short history, smoked rather than injected heroin use, low level of use, and good general motivation and social support.

Lofexidine need not be restricted to such cases, as a switch to this treatment may be effective in individuals who have difficulties in the later stages of a methadone reduction, and the drug is also useful in inpatient and custodial settings, where quick detoxification is indicated and there may be various problems in using methadone. Clonidine is now virtually confined to inpatient treatment, where hypotension can be monitored and some patients may actually value the sedative effect. The general desire for shorter admissions in inpatient treatment has led to the development of various experimental techniques, which may incorporate the precipitation of withdrawal by opiate antagonists, followed by symptomatic treatment under heavy sedation or even general anaesthetic.

A reducing course of methadone remains a standard approach for opiate detoxification in the UK, although elsewhere methadone is often considered only suitable for maintenance treatment. Certainly a methadone detoxification frequently appears to be an uncomfortable process, with prolonged and distressing withdrawal effects, but it is important to distinguish the difficulties which may arise from extent of previous dependence, the detoxification method itself, and the general adjustment to becoming drug free. Short-term methadone detoxification from street heroin is relatively well tolerated, with detoxification from established maintenance much more problematic, and so it would appear to be the general 'addictiveness' of methadone which ultimately produces problems in the withdrawal situation. The widely-held clinical impression that any withdrawal method is more comfortable if it is from heroin rather than from methadone is backed up by the limited systematic evidence, while it is notable that most studies of methadone detoxification courses lasting 10–21 days have been in the inpatient setting. Methadone detoxification in the community tends to be over much longer time periods, with a slow withdrawal over one to two years a common timescale. Candidates for this would often elsewhere be considered suitable for maintenance treatment, but a large proportion of patients in the UK elect to come off methadone even if ongoing treatment is available. Slow detoxification is often a tortuous process, and related practical management problems can be among the most time-consuming aspects of drug misuse treatment.

Methadone treatment is indicated in pregnant opiate misusers, due to the inadvisability of quick detoxification. A maintenance dose throughout pregnancy may be required in severely dependent individuals, but the balance of the neonatal evidence favours a full withdrawal from opiates if this is feasible for the mother. Various factors may conspire against early presentation of pregnant users, and the extent of methadone reduction depends partly on the time available, given that the rate has to be cautious. The opiate agonist–antagonist buprenorphine may in future prove to be a suitable treatment drug in pregnancy, and its properties suggest that it may prove preferable to methadone in detoxification treatment generally.

In our view naltrexone should be used routinely after opiate detoxification, given the high risk of relapse. An advantage of the nonopioid detoxification methods is that naltrexone can be started virtually straight after the medication course, without the wait that is necessary if methadone or even dihydrocodeine has been used. We present nonopioid detoxification and naltrexone treatment as essentially one package, and find not only that the acceptability of naltrexone is high, but that the prospect of having the medication is often one of the main motivations for treatment. A naloxone challenge or supervised first dose is necessary at the outset of naltrexone treatment, following which ongoing supervision of dosing by a family member or partner is highly desirable, as with disulfiram in alcohol misuse. Naltrexone should usually be continued for one to three months in the first instance, and then for as long as it seems to be required, with no evidence to suggest any particular set beneficial period. Associated relapse prevention counselling should address the characteristic difficulties which drug misusers face when initially attempting to live without drug taking.

# 4

## Treatment of nonopiate misuse

### Introduction

This book is mainly concerned with the treatment of opiate misuse, for the simple reason that that is the form of drug misuse for which there are the most effective clinical treatments. As we have discussed, the treatment scene for opiate misusers, in contrast to other groups, is fundamentally altered by the widespread availability of the substitution option, in the form of methadone or possibly alternative opioids. Physical dependence is part of the rationale for that approach, and the occurrence of clear-cut withdrawal symptoms also indicates the use of drugs such as lofexidine or clonidine, followed where possible by naltrexone. For reasons of severity of dependence and treatment options, it is therefore understandable that services are drawn to having caseloads dominated by opiate users.

This does not mean that there is nothing that can be done for other drug misusers, although that is the message which is sometimes conveyed. In the UK around the late 1980s there was a definite impression of helplessness regarding managing users of nonopiate drugs, which followed the large expansion of methadone prescribing services. Low-threshold prescribing had been advocated for opiate users at risk of HIV transmission, and the recently-formed community drug services were strongly encouraged to deliver such treatment, with counselling approaches becoming neglected. If amphetamine users or other groups then presented, the often openly-asked question was 'if we can't prescribe, what can we do with them?', and debates followed about the relative need for nonmedical and medical services. As indicated elsewhere, the prescribing ethos led to experimentation with that approach for some amphetamine users, but in a further process of development, general counselling skills now appear to be being rediscovered, ironically probably helped by the presentation of many newer heroin users who are suited to detoxification rather than to methadone. Clearly, the range of counselling skills are even more necessary in the treatment of nonopiate misuse, where there are precious few effective pharmacological treatment options.

General counselling for drug misusers is discussed in Chapter 5, and the particular approaches relating to the situations of detoxification and relapse prevention in Chapter 3. The more expertly a service can provide drug counselling, the more confident it can be in managing nonopiate misusers, and possibly even attracting such groups. Because use of amphetamines in particular, and also other recreational drugs, is so commonly a precursor to opiate use, this even raises a question regarding priorities for clinical services, for which there is no easy answer. Should services prioritize opiate users, because the treatments are most direct and effective, or could prioritizing at least the younger nonopiate users fulfil a preventive role, in that individuals would not then progress on to opiates? Counselling no doubt has to be very expert for the latter preventive effect to occur, while within limited budgets the opiate misusers should not be denied their more obvious treatment opportunities. The balance is a difficult one to strike, and for a community drug service this relates partly to the extent to which it has wide responsibility for the overall management of drug problems in its area, or a more specialized clinical role within a range of services.

In nonopiate misuse it is the specific clinical treatments, beyond harm reduction and counselling approaches, which are so limited, and this chapter will examine the evidence for effectiveness of such treatments for each form of drug misuse in turn.

## Cocaine

Most of our knowledge of treating cocaine misuse comes from the USA, following the massive epidemic of the problem there throughout the 1980s (Warner 1993). In the middle of that decade it was estimated that approximately one-tenth of the population had used cocaine, and while no other country is set to have an equivalent experience, severe cocaine-related problems are being encountered in many areas, including the UK's major cities. This is especially so now that cocaine is increasingly used in the 'crack' form, which is associated with generally higher levels of the various adverse effects and social complications. Some of the important features of this form of drug misuse are indicated in Table 4.1.

The transition from cocaine hydrochloride to crack has changed the face of cocaine usage. Claims used to be made for the hydrochloride as a harmless desirable accompaniment to the executive lifestyle and, apart

Table 4.1. *Important features of cocaine misuse*

Rise of 'crack' form, more addictive
Minority of users develop extreme usage
Often periodic
More medically dangerous than heroin
Psychotic features common
Various links with violent crime

from the well known complication of damage to the nasal septum from snorting the drug, millions of individuals no doubt have used cocaine powder with relatively few adverse effects. (The injected use by polydrug users, for instance in combination with heroin, is inherently much more hazardous.) Crack is produced from cocaine hydrochloride by a simple chemical process, and this purer, more volatile form is much more potent in its effects and withdrawal symptoms. Very rapid rises in blood levels of the drug are achieved by smoking, and this method, using various forms of apparatus, is the main route of administration, although habitual drug injectors will break crack down and inject it. Crack can be said to be more addictive, if that term is used to include the profound psychological features which occur rather than bodily withdrawal symptoms. In particular, craving and acute depressive feelings on withdrawal can be extremely severe, and partly account for the rapidly escalating usage of a minority of individuals. The extent to which individuals become 'hooked' is very variable with crack, and so while many can take the drug on an occasional basis without problems, others develop a compulsive, and indeed extreme, form of usage, spending vast amounts of money in short spaces of time. Fortunately, such usage is not sustainable, and an important feature of cocaine misuse is that it is often periodic, in contrast to the stereotyped daily routine of a dependent heroin user.

Because of cocaine's stimulant effects on the noradrenergic system, heavy use carries significant risks of cardiovascular complications, including myocardial infarction and stroke, with high rates of these seen in the USA epidemic (Cregler & Mark 1986, Galanter et al. 1992). Psychiatric effects are also common (Mendoza & Miller 1992), including paranoid psychosis which is well known among users; in heavy usage acute psychotic states can be severe and pose problems in containment of disturbed behaviour. Aggressiveness and violence frequently occur in such states and in other situations (Giannini et al. 1993), including craving for crack, when desperate measures may be adopted to obtain the drug. The crack dealing scene appears to be a particularly violent one, notably associated with gun crime, while crack misuse in women is strongly linked with prostitution, at least in the UK. Babies born to crack-using women may have specific abnormalities (Kain, Kain & Scarpelli 1992), and there is an increased risk of obstetric complications (Hulse et al. 1997).

As with other stimulant misusers, those who use cocaine will often also take various sedative drugs to terminate an episode of use and alleviate withdrawal effects. These have typically included cannabis, alcohol and benzodiazepines, but in the UK heroin is increasingly being taken for this purpose by crack users, sometimes to the point of becoming physically dependent on the opiate. The common stereotype used to be the crack user who is a dealer in heroin but never takes that drug himself, but in general it appears that these two forms of drug use are overlapping more, both within individuals and also subculturally.

The possible treatments for cocaine misuse and the evidence for their effectiveness have been the subject of several authoritative reviews from the USA (Rawson et al. 1991, Withers et al. 1995, Warner et al. 1997, Nathan et al. 1998). A large number of pharmacological treatments have been tried, with other interest focused on various types of residential programmes, cognitive and behavioural approaches, and alternative therapies such as acupuncture. These will be examined briefly from the perspective of a particular interest I have in cocaine misuse treatment, having been involved in the main investigation so far of treatment in the UK (Donmall et al. 1995), and facing a substantial crack scene in Sheffield.

**Pharmacological treatments**
We observed earlier that the main treatment in opiate misuse, methadone, can be seen broadly as a substitution approach, offering direct relief of withdrawal symptoms and various other medical and social benefits. There is currently no real consideration of that model of treatment in cocaine misuse, although both methylphenidate and amphetamine have previously been used in limited experiments along those lines. In general, the arguments against cocaine prescribing are considered to be the same as those which weigh against widespread acceptance of amphetamine prescribing (see page 65), but applying even more so, especially the aspect of adverse effects of the drug itself.

Instead, investigations have mainly been of medications which may alleviate cocaine withdrawal features by less direct mechanisms (Withers et al. 1995, Warner et al. 1997, Nathan et al. 1998). The classic description of cocaine withdrawal (Gawin & Kleber 1986) identifies a syndrome in three stages: initially agitation, anorexia and acute craving; secondly excessive tiredness, depression and hyperphagia; and finally a normalization of most features but a return of craving when triggered by environmental cues. The euphoria produced by cocaine and the prominent withdrawal features of craving and depression are considered to be largely due to an increase, and then rebound depletion, in central dopamine transmission, and most early interest was in the dopaminergic drugs bromocriptine and amantadine, and the antidepressant desipramine which acts substantially on dopamine transmission (Pollack, Brotman & Rosenbaum 1989). Controlled studies have mainly been of desipramine, with a meta-analysis indicating benefit over placebo in promoting abstinence, but not in treatment retention (Levin & Lehman 1991). To varying degrees, these three medications tend to be poorly tolerated, and studies continue to produce mixed results (Warner et al. 1997). Carbamazepine has also been advocated (Halikas et al. 1992), on the basis that the withdrawal symptoms may represent minor convulsive phenomena, but controlled studies have not supported use of the drug (Montoya et al. 1995).

An alternative approach with antidepressants is to use the specific serotonergic re-uptake inhibitors such as fluoxetine (Covi et al. 1995). Serotonin transmission is affected by cocaine in similar ways to that of dopamine (Benowitz 1992), while other rationales for the use of these medications include quicker onset of action than the tricyclics, better acceptability, plus a possible effect in reducing drug craving which has been indicated in animal studies (Sellers et al. 1991) and in some amphetamine users (see page 129). Once again, however, there is little supporting evidence (Grabowski et al. 1995), and with lithium and antipsychotic drugs also having been tried as treatments, there is no doubt much truth in the observation that the large number of drugs which have been investigated in cocaine misuse is testament to the fact that none of them have very good effect. Certainly in states of heavy compulsive crack use the prospects of medication making a significant impression can seem slight, sometimes with the exception of sedative antipsychotic drugs for agitation. In the presence of definite psychotic symptoms full doses of a suitable antipsychotic may be required for a period, combined with efforts to prevent ongoing cocaine use. Benzodiazepines also have a limited role as symptomatic treatment in the acute stages of withdrawal (see page 72).

## Nonpharmacological treatments

Residential programmes and relapse prevention work for cocaine mis-users often represent modified forms of treatment that is applicable across all substances (Rawson et al. 1991, Zweben 1986). On a visit to a USA treatment centre as background to our own cocaine research I remember receiving in response to the question 'what works for cocaine misuse?', the answer 'alcohol treatment'. Certainly both groups are required to work towards total abstinence from their drug, and similar strategies can be brought to bear in individual and group therapies, while experienced units also take into account sub-cultural differences between the users of various drugs.

One reasonably well recognized specific feature of cocaine use is that withdrawal craving, and therefore risk of relapse, appears to be strongly 'cue-dependent' (Weddington et al. 1990). Thus, an individual may ex-perience relatively few problems staying abstinent from cocaine in the early stages, until he or she encounters the particular situation in which they formerly used cocaine, when high arousal and strong cravings can occur. This makes an inpatient setting generally unrealistic for relapse prevention work, but in some units experimental situations have been set up where cues are simulated or drug paraphernalia presented, to work on the process of habituation (O'Brien et al. 1990). A very different behav-ioural approach was used in community patients by Higgins et al. (1994a), who gave material incentives (retail vouchers) as rewards for cocaine-free urines. In a controlled trial the scheme showed benefits additional to those of the general counselling treatment, and there has been a good deal of interest in the findings, although applicability would no doubt vary in different settings. There is some evidence in favour of coping skills training, a technique involving the analysis and practice of skills required in avoiding relapse, preferably focusing specifically on cocaine problems (Monti et al. 1997). It might be felt that such an approach would only be suitable in relatively straightforward cases, but the authors point out that in their work with alcoholics the technique was particularly effective in those with higher levels of sociopathy or psychopathology.

In the wide-ranging search for treatments for cocaine misuse, alterna-tive therapies have been tried, with one controlled study showing a limited benefit of acupuncture over 'placebo' acupuncture (i.e. placing the needles in sites not previously recognized as acting on drug with-drawal symptoms) (Lipton et al. 1994).

**Additional findings from studies**

There are various findings in the range of studies suggesting additional factors which may be relevant in the provision of treatment. Adverse outcomes have been found with some personality characteristics, namely 'manipulative, exploitive and confrontive interpersonal features' (McMahon et al. 1993), and DSM-III antisocial personality disorder (Arndt et al. 1994), therefore according with findings in other forms of drug misuse (Seivewright & Daly 1997). Additional depression might similarly be expected to have an adverse effect on prognosis but, on the other hand, antidepressants are a common form of treatment in cocaine misuse, and so depressed patients might actually show greater improvements overall. In one randomized controlled trial in cocaine-misusing methadone-maintenance patients, the choice of treatment appeared relevant in this way, with depression actually a good prognostic factor in those who received medication including desipramine, but a poor prognostic factor in others (Ziedonis & Kosten 1991). In terms of gender, females have been demonstrated to have better six-month outcome than males following pharmacological treatment for cocaine misuse, despite having more severe drug problems at intake (Kosten et al. 1993).

The subject of features of treatment programmes which have beneficial effects on outcome has been reviewed by Khalsa et al. (1993). Characteristics of treatment which tended to improve retention rates and outcomes were identified as frequent group therapy, individual and family therapy, intensive structuring of programmes, cocaine-specific education, supervised urine testing, and encouragement to use self-help groups. However, the difficulties of comparing across very different types of treatment were emphasized, and the findings could not be considered conclusive. Higgins et al. (1994b) ventured a preliminary finding that the single best predictor of cocaine abstinence during outpatient behavioural treatment for cocaine dependence was whether a 'significant other' participated in treatment.

**Deployment of treatments**

In the UK we have been in a somewhat expectant position in the past few years, waiting to see the extent to which crack misuse would cross the Atlantic, and the problems which would result. So far, our experience appears to be similar to that of Australia, as described by Hando et al. (1997), although we are different in terms of population demographics, ethnic groups and international networks. In both countries the rates of presentation of primary users of cocaine or crack to treatment services is

Table 4.2. *Themes in treatment of cocaine misuse in England*

| |
|---|
| Specific outreach |
| Prioritization |
| Practical counselling |
| Targeted use of pharmacological treatments |
| Admission in some severe cases |
| Acupuncture commonly used |

Based on Donmall et al. (1995)

low, in comparison with the dominance of opiate users receiving methadone, but most indicators show a steady increase in cocaine availability and use by inner-city polydrug users. In a recent project we were interested to investigate which treatments are given in the UK to cocaine misusers who do present, since it is clear from the literature that there is no consensus of opinion to support strongly any single treatment, or even range of treatments.

In a three-stage investigation (Donmall et al. 1995) we carried out a survey of drug misuse treatment services in England, then interviewed staff at services which were seeing relatively large numbers of cocaine misusers, and studied a cohort of patients in treatment. Among a wide range of findings, some common themes emerged which were considered important in the treatment of cocaine misusers by workers across the range of disciplines. These are indicated in Table 4.2.

These aspects of the deployment of treatments clearly do not represent definitive guidance – in a way they are rather the opposite, having developed in real-life clinical situations in the absence of much directly relevant research evidence. They are useful, however, in the consideration of how to engage and manage cocaine misusers successfully in a community drug service.

It was widely observed that cocaine users are not inclined to attend services as they are delivered at present, and there had been various initiatives to outreach to specific groups, including Afro-Caribbean people and women. Often, cocaine users were given priority appointments, since attendance from a waiting list tended to be poor, one factor perhaps being the periodicity of usage. Where engagement was successful, counselling was mainly of a very practical nature, addressing immediate lifestyle problems and offering basic advice on harm reduction and methods of cutting down. Pharmacological treatments were used by nearly half of the services which offered any treatment, with a wide range of medications directed at various features of cocaine usage. Fluoxetine and desipramine were the most frequently prescribed antidepressants, with benzodiazepines used to aid sleep and reduce agitation in withdrawal states. Thioridazine was the most selected antipsychotic drug, apparently because of its general sedative effect as well as for use in direct treatment of psychotic complications. Most staff we interviewed had had experience of crack users presenting in states of heavy compulsive usage and great distress, such that admission of some kind was considered the only feasible option. Signs of physical or psychiatric illness would indicate hospital settings, but some rehabilitation centres accepted individuals whose main need appeared to be simply removal from availability of crack. The recourse to admission in acute situations highlighted the dearth of treatments definitely effective in reducing cocaine use, as in a different way did the generally widespread use of acupuncture and other alternative therapies.

Our research was the first substantially to investigate clinical treatments in England, and in general confirmed the perceived limitations of specific treatments in cocaine misuse. It was instructive, however, to see the approaches of those projects, often outside the statutory sector, which were positively directed at engaging this group, who are only seen in small numbers by most services. Specific outreach of various kinds appeared essential, to counteract the commonly held view that drug services mainly exist to give methadone to male white heroin users. At the start of this chapter it was acknowledged that clinical services need to concentrate their efforts on substantially managing opiate misuse, as being the most amenable to treatment, but in areas of high cocaine prevalence there must also be some facility to develop treatment options for users of this drug, given the severity of problems which can occur.

### Cocaine misuse by methadone patients

One form of cocaine misuse which is encountered frequently in services is the additional use of the drug by patients on methadone. Cocaine use at entry to programmes or during treatment has been extremely common in the USA (Magura et al. 1994), while the extent to which it is seen in methadone clinics in the UK largely depends on local availability. In some ways cocaine is a particularly appealing drug to use along with methadone, as a 'speed ball' effect can be had from the combination (whereas heroin's effects are often reduced by methadone), and there is no risk of increasing opiate tolerance. Chaisson et al. (1989) found that 24% of cocaine users whom they studied began or increased cocaine injection following entry into a methadone treatment programme.

Methadone treatment under 'contract' generally requires abstinence from other drugs, and so to some extent elimination of cocaine use ought to be achieved simply be enforcing the rules of the programme. In formal terms this can be called 'contingency management', and structured versions of this approach, sometimes with rewards, have been applied to adjunctive use of cocaine, as well as to other drugs such as benzodiazepines. The approach of giving retail vouchers for cocaine-free urines, mentioned above in primary users, has also been successful in cocaine-misusing methadone patients (Silverman et al. 1996). Another nonspecific approach to the problem is to consider increasing methadone dose, if it appears that an individual is supplementing with cocaine because of perceived inadequate maintenance effect.

The evidence relating to various strategies in cocaine-misusing methadone patients has been reviewed by Rawson et al. (1994). In terms of pharmacological treatments, several of the same drugs have been tried in this group as in primary cocaine misusers, with limited success. A report of fluoxetine being effective in a series of cases (Pollack & Rosenbaum 1991) was not supported by a placebo-controlled double-blind trial (Grabowski et al. 1995). An alternative pharmacological strategy has been to change the opioid maintenance agent from methadone to the partial agonist buprenorphine, partly based on the possibility that the reinforcing 'speedball' effects may be less (Foltin & Fischman 1996). Once again, however, benefits were not demonstrated in a controlled study (Strain et al. 1994b). The review of treatments (Rawson et al. 1994) includes some practical suggestions on reducing the risk of crack dealing around a clinic, and on running groups specifically for those methadone patients who have problems with cocaine.

As indicated earlier, a minority of the crack users in the UK who use heroin to 'come down' from their drug become dependent enough on the opiate for methadone to be considered. In such cases of true dual dependency, methadone may offer the best chance of a stabilizing effect on drug use and lifestyle, but the same rules of treatment need to be applied as to any other methadone patient. In practice, progress in those who were primarily crack users tends to be problematic, with difficulties in abstaining from the favoured drug, and often poor acceptance of methadone's effects. Further expertise needs to be gained with this group, and the situation must be avoided whereby methadone is simply offering an alternative sedative to those previously used, with little impact on stimulant use.

**Case history**

Darren is a 26-year-old man who was referred to our clinic as having problems with heroin and cocaine use. He was on probation following offences of robbery and assault, and a preliminary discussion with his probation officer indicated that crack cocaine had originally been Darren's drug of preference. His offences were related to his use of crack, at a time when he had been spending large amounts of money on the drug. Heroin use had gradually developed over the past year, and at two assessment appointments there were clinical signs of heroin use, and both drugs present in the urine.

The situation of daily dependent heroin use was sufficient to merit methadone treatment, but a detoxification attempt was not successful. His initial dosage was reinstated and the urine tests at his further appointments did not show heroin, but four consecutive tests showed cocaine, benzodiazepines and cannabis, in addition to his methadone. It was explained to Darren that we would need to discharge him from methadone treatment by reducing the course quickly, and he had no major complaints.

Darren had also made contacts with a local street agency aimed at crack users, and he continued to see them frequently. Our next involvement was when we were asked to assess him in relation to funding for a stay at an out-of-town residential rehabilitation centre. It transpired that his situation had improved substantially, with a general reduction in drug use and temporary employment gained through a probation scheme. He claimed to no longer use opiates, but he would occasionally obtain tranquillizers and he sometimes drank heavily. He had made personal efforts, with support, to greatly reduce his use of crack, but he experienced strong cravings, and his mood was frequently low. There were clinical grounds for prescribing an antidepressant, and he was given fluoxetine 20 mg per day, and reviewed at a short series of appointments. He reports some reduction in craving and improvement in mood, and urine sampling accords with his self-reported reductions in drug use. He was approved for residential treatment, but at present he does not wish to take this up because of his job, and because he feels he can manage without it.

## Amphetamine

There is an extraordinary lack of literature on the treatment of amphetamine problems, with this subject almost universally regarded by observers of treatment in the UK as an unjustly neglected area. Use of the drug is hugely widespread but, as with cocaine, voluntary presentation to services other than needle exchange is at a very low rate. Amphetamine misuse does not have the same high media profile as that of cocaine, and yet the reasons for which services were exhorted to engage large numbers of drug users at the time of the HIV crisis would appear to be particularly pertinent to this group. These frustrations have been well voiced by Klee (1992), who refers to amphetamine use as 'a case study in neglect', in which the 'myopic focus on the casualties of heroin' has led to amphetamine problems 'not being taken seriously'. She presents comparative data showing higher rates of HIV risk-taking behaviours in injecting amphetamine users than heroin users, and points to the many studies indicating high levels of sexual activity.

With studies of treatment few and far between, the general forms of management have been discussed from a UK perspective by ourselves (Seivewright & McMahon 1996), and by Myles (1997). The use of harm-reduction measures, general and specialized counselling, and pharmacological treatments for withdrawal features or psychiatric complications, may be seen as basically similar to the application of the same approaches in cocaine misuse, while in drug services there has been interest in two particular treatment aspects. In a series of cases Polson et al. (1993) found that fluoxetine, in ordinary dosage of 20 mg per day, helped some amphetamine users cut down or stop their drug. The medication was given for two weeks in the first instance, with counselling therapies where indicated. This evidence is basically no stronger than that for the same treatment in cocaine misuse, but in the absence of controlled trials of *any* treatment, the strategy has been quite widely taken up by services which see significant numbers of amphetamine users. Given the other evidence for serotonergic re-uptake inhibitors reducing drug craving and appetitive and compulsive behaviours (Sellers et al. 1991), it certainly seems reasonable to select a medication of this type if significant persistent depression in a stimulant user suggests an antidepressant. The second treatment approach which is being used is more controversial, namely limited substitute prescribing with dexamphetamine sulphate (Bradbeer et al. 1998). Many specialists in the UK consider that, although a substitution approach is inherently much less satisfactory in amphetamine users than opiate users for various reasons, it is not necessary to rule it out completely, and will prescribe in some cases of severe dependence. This issue is discussed in detail in Chapter 2.

The treatment options for amphetamine users in our own community services, which have developed pragmatically over a number of years, are summarized in Table 4.3.

Most amphetamine users purely receive drug counselling, covering the

Table 4.3. *A scheme for community treatment of amphetamine misuse*

| Treatment | Indications |
|---|---|
| Counselling alone | Short-term use ( < 6 months)<br>Occasional use<br>Not injecting |
| Counselling plus limited course of symptomatic medication: fluoxetine, diazepam, nitrazepam | Inability to otherwise tolerate withdrawal effects |
| Counselling plus dexamphetamine sulphate prescribing | Heavy daily injected use<br>Severe direct health or social problems<br>Other approaches failed but motivation to avoid illicit amphetamine is high |

aspects described in the section on general counselling in Chapter 5. This includes all individuals whose amphetamine use is short term and/or occasional (e.g. weekends), and those in whom there is no convincing indication for pharmacological treatments. Nearly all such users take the street powder form (commonly about 5% pure), by ingestion or snorting. Beyond simply weekend use, other users take the drug for a run of a few days, until some over-agitation and paranoid experiences signal the time to stop and catch up on eating and sleeping. In counselling, such users are specifically encouraged to increase their drug-free days, and advised on behavioural tactics which can help in doing this.

The next category of treatment comprises drug counselling plus symptomatic medication, and is for those who want to stop their usage but have found themselves unable to do so through not being able to tolerate the withdrawal effects. Many such individuals use amphetamine on most days, and they may have progressed to injecting. Amphetamine withdrawal features are usually considered to primarily include depression, hypersomnia and hyperphagia, with debate as to whether such features constitute a syndrome as such, or whether they simply represent the rebound effects of the drug's actions. Many relatively heavy users who attempt to stop, however, experience a more complex combination of symptoms: irritability and aggressiveness are frequent and may partly represent a personality-determined response to discomfort, while there are often various aches and pains, anxiety and craving, with insomnia occurring after two or three days if the withdrawal attempt lasts that far. In a well motivated individual who has experienced such difficulties, we prescribe diazepam and nitrazepam in moderate dosage in a one to two week course, plus fluoxetine 20 mg per day. Such prescribing is satisfactory only if it is part of a concentrated and supported effort to abstain, but with good community supervision the alleviation of symptoms, notably insomnia, can enable successful withdrawal. Benzodiazepines must be clearly time-limited to avoid dependence, but fluoxetine may be continued for the length of a normal antidepressant course if there are convincing clinical grounds.

Prescribing of dexamphetamine sulphate is considered only in the most severe cases of dependence, such as individuals using in the order of 7 grams per day, injecting several times a day, often with a history dating back many years. There must not only be demonstrable severe health or social problems produced by such use, but the individual must be motivated to greatly modify or preferably stop their use of street amphetamine if taken on for prescribing. Like other services, although we would much rather always prescribe on the basis of complete abstinence, we have had cases where intravenous use is so heavy that prescribing has been effectively on harm-reduction grounds. General criteria, monitoring and prescribing methods are as described in Chapter 2, where there is a case history from our service. At the levels of street amphetamine usage for which we prescribe, a starting dose of 60 mg per day of dexamphetamine sulphate mixture is usually required; this is considered a maximum, so that if prescribing were done, exceptionally for a person using only 2–3 grams per day, the daily dexamphetamine dose could be 40 mg. Dispensing is two to three times per week, with gradual reductions in daily dosage and/or in the number of days on which medication is taken in a week. We prescribe for a maximum of six months, and so the aim is for full reduction during this time. When prescribing is purely on a harm-reduction basis, the same maximum period is applied, in which case repeat courses may be necessary after a period, with the user strongly encouraged to move towards reduction and abstinence.

Many drug services in the UK are providing treatment for amphetamine users along similar lines to the above scheme at the present time. Systematic and assertive drug counselling should be the basis of treatment, and where efforts are directed at engaging more amphetamine users, it should primarily be with that aim and to provide the direct harm-reduction measures such as injecting equipment provision. The prescribing element attracts the controversy, and is sometimes over-emphasized in terms of promoting engagement, but in the present state of evidence this can only be considered suitable for an extremely small proportion of cases.

### Case history

Robert is 28 years old and had used drugs since teenage years. For many years his preference was amphetamines, progressing to daily injected use. He then moved on to using heroin, presenting to our service about a year later. He did a successful community detoxification from heroin but, perhaps predictably, re-lapsed into amphetamine use. He was re-referred by the probation service after committing several offences.

At this time Robert was injecting amphetamine several times a day, and was living in a house with several other amphetamine users. He had clearly become paranoid, believing the television was referring to him, and generally avoiding people.

The drug worker who knew Robert from before took on his case, and saw him for a series of appointments. Counselling emphasized that the time was right to give up amphetamine, as his family had become very concerned and were willing to support him. He was helped to become aware that amphetamine was causing his mental symptoms, and he was systematically encouraged to have drug-free days, on an increasing basis.

In just three weeks Robert stopped using amphetamine, with no medication necessary. In view of the progress he had made, he was given support and assistance in finding accommodation of his own. His paranoid symptoms resolved, to the extent that he volunteered information to the police to clear up some previous charges. Three months on, there has been no relapse and no new offending behaviour.

## Methylenedioxymethamphetamine (MDMA, 'ecstasy')

This is the drug which has had such a strong influence in the nightclub culture in the UK and elsewhere through the 1990s. With semihal-lucinogenic effects in addition to the stimulant amphetamine actions, it has been associated with a revival of 'psychedelia', to some extent recalling the use of LSD in the 1960s. The distinctive modern setting for using ecstasy, however, is at a 'rave', typically all-night, with characteris-tic repetitive and energetic music and dancing. Taking ecstasy or an alternative stimulant or hallucinogen is almost an integral part of the rave experience (Boys et al. 1997), and in youth culture in the UK this has represented the most significant new wave of drug taking since the advent of smokable heroin. Amphetamine and LSD are commonly used by the same individuals and groups, while there are many slight chemical variants of ecstasy, such as methylenedioxyethylamphetamine (MDEA, 'eve'), and unrelated chemicals are sometimes marketed as ecstasy, such as ketamine.

Ecstasy tablets can be taken in various different individual situations apart from at raves, but in general the modern usage appears characterized by higher doses and/or more frequent consumption than were typical in a previous era of recreational use in the USA (Peroutka et al. 1988). That earlier usage owed something to a legal (at the time) use in psychotherapy, and appears to have been generally fairly restrained, although widespread, particularly among college students. Alongside the desired effects, a range of minor adverse effects were recognized, some of which resembled those of amphetamine, including anorexia, and irritability and depression on stopping the drug. Some were slightly more characteristic, such as jaw tension and teeth grinding, but the major problems have only emerged as usage has become generally heavier and associated with the nightclub scene.

The most severe adverse effects are unexpected deaths and a range of psychiatric complications, and in both cases there is a limited understanding of aetiology (Solowij 1993, Ghodse & Kreek 1997). The sudden deaths have often followed the development of hyperthermia, with features such as disseminated intravascular coagulation, rhabdomyolysis and acute renal failure (Henry et al. 1992). Dosage in these individual instances seems of limited relevance, with some deaths having occurred after just one tablet, and the hot environmental conditions in nightclubs have been implicated. Spontaneous intracerebral haemorrhage has also been reported, while of the nonfatal complications, a toxic hepatitis may relate partly to contaminants (Solowij 1993).

The connection between ecstasy use and a range of alleged psychiatric adverse effects is difficult to ascertain. Beyond the minor depressive reactions which are common after stimulants (and can cause absenteeism after weekend ecstasy use), other conditions which appear possible complications include anxiety and panic disorders, more severe depression, psychoses and flashback experiences. On the one hand, the scattering of case reports in the literature are somewhat unconvincing, often with confounding factors such as other drug use or family history of psychosis (Solowij 1993), but other community research (Williamson et al. 1997) and clinical experience suggest quite strong links. Pre-existing vulnerability to psychiatric or physical conditions is often suggested as an explanation of why only a small proportion of users suffer ill effects, but there are also striking reports of panic disorder (McCann & Ricaurte 1992) and catatonic stupor (Maxwell et al. 1993) occurring in previously healthy individuals after single doses of the drug. In general, it may be relevant that ecstasy and related compounds are known to be neurotoxic to serotonergic neurones in various animals including primates (Fischer et al. 1995), but the significance of associated abnormalities which have been demonstrated in humans (McCann et al. 1994) is as yet uncertain. In a post mortem study, a range of neuropathological changes in the brain have been demonstrated, along with various organ toxicity effects, in individuals who had taken ecstasy or MDEA (Milroy et al. 1996).

With ecstasy users rarely presenting to treatment services other than after the development of complications, the management of this form of drug misuse has mainly been in the harm-reduction arena. Because dehydration appears important in the potentially fatal physical effects, there has been much advice for users at raves regarding measures such as taking rest periods and maintaining an adequate fluid intake, with organizers being required to make suitable conditions available. Unfortunately the perils of giving advice of this kind have been brought home by the knowledge that some deaths have involved dilutional effects of over-hydration, which has left the harm-reduction situation in some confusion. It seems that the recommendations regarding amounts of fluid to drink have been broadly correct, but that some individuals may develop a kind of compulsive drinking, which it is known can occur with amphetamine misuse.

Treatment of psychiatric complications should generally be along standard lines for the respective conditions. Some syndromes appear to be brief and self-limiting once ecstasy use stops, but a more chronic course may also be seen, with cases in the literature of psychoses which prove resistant to treatment (Solowij 1993). Whichever psychiatric syndrome occurs, there is possibly a theoretical indication for specific serotonergic re-uptake inhibitors such as fluoxetine, given the effect of ecstasy in reducing serotonin transmission. This would purely be a pragmatic approach which has not yet been formally tested, and it may be that the transmission abnormalities are not amenable to this kind of enhancement.

### Case history

Paul was referred by his general practitioner to our clinic, at 29 years old with no previous contact. He was a successful business man, and lived in a desirable residential area with his parents. He drank alcohol in moderation, and until recently his only drug use was smoking cannabis on a handful of occasions.

Two months before presenting to his doctor, Paul had used ecstasy twice at a nightclub, about a week apart. He reported that he had 'not felt right since', experiencing anxiety and some more severe panic attacks. He had been unable to concentrate at work, and generally felt he was functioning poorly. He had palpitations on any significant exertion, and had little energy. Over the period he had felt increasingly depressed, wondering what was happening to him and sometimes breaking down in tears. His appetite was poor and he had lost some weight.

It was considered that his symptoms could be directly due to ecstasy, but also that some secondary anxiety and depression were likely. For short-term symptom relief he was prescribed diazepam 2 mg tablets up to four per day for one week. He was also given fluoxetine 20 mg per day, and the need to avoid ecstasy or any illicit drugs was reinforced.

Paul's various symptoms improved slowly over the course of about three months. Sometimes his anxiety would become more prominent, and very limited further supplies of diazepam were given. The improvement in mood was also not dramatic, with the effect of medication uncertain. He is now on no medication, and feels virtually back to his 'old self'. He is sure that he will not use ecstasy or any other drugs again and, with the increased risk through anxiety, he has been advised not to increase his alcohol intake.

## Benzodiazepines

Benzodiazepine problems are typically thought of as relating to individuals with minor psychiatric disorders, literally millions of whom have become dependent after being prescribed the drugs in ordinary dosage (Lader 1993). Clear-cut demonstrations of physical dependence in controlled studies occurred some two decades after the drugs had been introduced (Tyrer et al. 1981, Petursson & Lader 1981), and there has been much criticism in retrospect of the over-prescribing of benzodiazepines in situations such as adjustment reactions or bereavement, and now also of the lack of treatment services for this group. Individuals dependent on prescribed benzodiazepines are reluctant to attend drug misuse services with their emphasis on illicit drug use, injecting and HIV, although some such services have separate support groups. Much of the management of benzodiazepine withdrawal takes place in primary care practice, and the usual approach, comprising preparation, transfer to a long-acting benzodiazepine, graded withdrawal, and additional counselling or pharmacological treatments, has been described in practical reviews (Lader & Morton 1991, Mant & Walsh 1997).

While some individuals who are prescribed benzodiazepines in ordinary circumstances increase their dosage to develop a form of definite misuse (Griffiths & Weerts 1997), the problems of benzodiazepine misuse by polydrug users are often very different in nature, as reviewed from the UK (Strang et al. 1993, Seivewright 1998), Australia (Darke 1994), and the USA (Griffiths & Weerts 1997). Studies have mainly been of prevalence and patterns of misuse, usually carried out in drug treatment settings such as methadone clinics, but with little examination of management of benzodiazepine misuse itself. Diazepam has been shown to enhance the subjective effects of opiates (Preston et al. 1984), and in one clinical survey most methadone maintenance patients who used diazepam reportedly took it within an hour of taking their methadone, for that reason (Stitzer et al. 1981). Benzodiazepines are also commonly taken by stimulant misusers (Darke et al. 1994a), partly to alleviate stimulant withdrawal effects, and by drug misusers with a preference for the similar effects of alcohol, or they may be a primary drug of misuse, relatively rarely in terms of presentation to treatment services. Prevalence rates of benzodiazepine use in polydrug users have been found to range up to 94% for lifetime use (Iguchi et al. 1993, Ross et al. 1997), with rates in studies largely determined by timescale and type of population investigated (Seivewright et al. 1993).

In the UK there has been particular concern over injected benzodiazepine misuse, usually of temazepam, which in the 1980s was formulated as a capsule with liquid content which could be extracted. This form of drug misuse produced severe psychological consequences such as amnesia and disturbed or aggressive behaviour (Ruben & Morrison 1992), and direct complications of injection leading to amputations have been frequent. The formulation was changed to a thicker gel content, but allegations followed that this had made matters worse, in that if drug misusers persisted in injecting temazepam the local effects seemed more severe. This was not clearly proved, but the drug has now been assigned to a higher level of control than the other benzodiazepines in the UK, and its prescription to drug misusers is generally discouraged. Because of the continued association of temazepam, even in tablet form, with high dose and injected misuse, in our own clinics we will not include this particular benzodiazepine in any of our prescribing regimes (see Chapter 2).

The temazepam phenomenon is an example of a very harmful form of benzodiazepine use by illicit drug users, but we may presume that overall there is a wide spectrum of harmfulness of usage with, at the lower end, occasional moderate oral use which may be unproblematic. Nevertheless, Darke and colleagues (Darke et al. 1992b, 1993, 1994a) found benzodiazepine use in polydrug users to be associated with a range of adverse physical, psychological and social features, suggesting both problems of a direct nature and also perhaps that benzodiazepine use may generally be an indicator of more severe drug misuse. One of the features consistently detected was increased HIV-risk behaviours, which fits with a study in which temazepam use was found to be strongly associated with a range of high-risk injecting and sexual practices (Klee et al. 1990). The possible explanations there appeared to be that either individuals who indulged in risky behaviours were selectively attracted to temazepam, or that some result of taking temazepam, such as the amnesia or confusion, produced the high-risk practices. That study was carried out at the height of the period of injected temazepam abuse in the UK, and links with HIV-risk behaviours cannot be assumed for all forms of benzodiazepine usage.

The most direct form of treatment of benzodiazepine misuse, deriving from the literature on ordinary-dose dependence, is detoxification where indicated, and this has been discussed in Chapter 2. Also in Chapters 1 and 2 there were extensive discussions of the difficulties which some methadone patients have in adjusting to that drug, and the need to sometimes use alternative substitutes. In this context, Ruben & Morrison (1992) suggested anecdotally that some of their patients who abused temazepam, apparently to boost the effects of methadone, were able to stop this when their methadone was changed to the injectable form. The inherently unsatisfactory option of offering some controlled benzodiazepine prescribing has also been discussed, while the preferable outcome in methadone patients would manifestly be able to eliminate benzodiazepine misuse by some additional intervention. Stitzer et al. (1982) reported some success with the use of 'contingency management', in which methadone patients were rewarded for benzodiazepine-free urines in the form of money, an increased dose of methadone, or take-home methadone. The study is a good example of both the limited applicability of techniques across different approaches to methadone treatment – since the method could only really operate in a fairly restrictive programme – and also of the paradoxical situations which relate to different forms of prescribing. It can readily be seen that any of the rewards could produce as destabilizing a situation as the benzodiazepine use which they are designed to eliminate, but nevertheless the broad principle is the important one of working within treatment contracts to shape other drug-taking behaviour. All such management is more likely to succeed in individuals who strongly wish to retain their methadone, and to a certain extent this has to be fostered.

## Cyclizine

Misuse of the antiemetic medication, cyclizine, is a rare form of drug misuse in overall terms, but for those of us in areas where it is prevalent it is extremely problematic. Following case reports of misuse by young people and pain patients, the first report of systematic misuse by illicit drug users (McLean & Casey 1982) and the only published study in such individuals so far (Ruben et al. 1989) were both from the city of Nottingham. Since then one of the doctors in our own clinic has also studied this form of usage closely (McMahon, unpublished data).

Cyclizine has antihistaminic, antiserotonic, local anaesthetic and vagolytic actions, and is marketed as a medication for vertigo and travel sickness. It is available without prescription although, since misuse has become recognized, its sale is at pharmacists' discretion. Cyclizine is a constituent, with the opioid dipipanone, in Diconal, and it appears to have opiate-enhancing effects which probably partly account for the marked popularity of Diconal among drug misusers.

Ruben et al. (1989) observed that cyclizine was appearing in the urine of the methadone patients in their clinic with increasing regularity, and interviewed 20 individuals who were identified as regular users, about their practices with the drug. This group misused cyclizine by injecting the crushed tablets, in varying doses but usually along with methadone. If patients were prescribed methadone mixture, they would typically attempt to obtain methadone tablets instead in order to inject the combination. The desired effects were stimulation, hallucinations, and to enhance the effect of methadone. The last was a recurring theme among the cases, with the summarized comments from individuals including 'need it to boost methadone', 'methadone no good without it', and 'methadone boring on its own'. After using cyclizine, the common reported effects were irritability, depression, aggressiveness and a strong craving for more of the drug. Four patients were said to have had epileptic fits.

In seeing patients in our methadone clinic almost daily who have misused cyclizine, we gain the impression of two kinds of usage. Some individuals inject the drug on its own, often in very large amounts and clearly seeking an intense effect. This may be repeated at closely-spaced intervals, until they become too confused to inject further, or lapse into unconsciousness. The other usage is more regular and controlled, and is common in long-term injectors who have a history of using Diconal but are now on injectable methadone. They will crush up, say, four or five cyclizine tablets and combine them with their methadone injection, to gain the enhanced opiate effect. We will not now prescribe methadone tablets because of the likelihood that they will be misused by injection, and McMahon (unpublished data) found that this was indeed occurring in all the cyclizine users he interviewed who were obtaining methadone tablets. His study included a nonclinic sample, who were attenders at a needle exchange, but most were obtaining methadone or injectable ampoules from other sources, and indeed cyclizine misuse appears inextricably linked with the use of methadone. From the accounts so far, it also appears that cyclizine is usually (possibly always) injected by drug misusers, and certainly if a methadone patient claims to be taking it orally this would be extremely unlikely. Misuse of benzodiazepines, particularly temazepam, also seems to be strongly associated with cyclizine use, and benzodiazepines should not be prescribed to such patients because of the risks of combined usage.

There is no information on management of this form of drug misuse. Of the usages described here, the elimination of the first, more chaotic, type of cyclizine usage would rely on general methods which address polydrug use. The only suggestion of a specific tactic could be in the second type of usage, where methadone patients are attempting to enhance the effects of that drug. For some such individuals who are manifestly unable to adjust to the stabilizing effects of methadone alone, there could possibly be benefit in prescribing an alternative opioid such as diamorphine, or alternatively even Cyclimorphine, to include a lesser controlled supply of cyclizine to intractable users. The latter can be strongly requested by patients who wish to avoid injecting crushed-up tablets, but clearly the situation is very open to abuse and, with cyclizine present in the urine, it is not possible to know whether additional supplies are being used. The problematic aspects of prescribing these two alternative drugs and other euphoriant opioids are discussed in detail in the first part of Chapter 2.

## Hallucinogens

Hallucinogenic mushrooms, containing psilocybin, and lysergic acid diethylamide (LSD) are extremely common recreational drugs. Like ecstasy and related drugs, LSD has a strong affinity at various types of serotonin receptors in the brain, and it is conceivable that serotonergic compounds could have some role in modifying the effects of LSD (O'Brien 1996). In practice, the times these forms of drug misuse are encountered by clinical services are when there are additional mental effects, such as acute confusional states, anxiety reactions or psychotic features. Hallucinogens may worsen preexisting mental disorders, and the implications in relation to psychoses are discussed in Chapter 8. There is particular debate about the status of 'flashback experiences', unwanted recurrences of drug effects which appear to occur for some time after use of LSD, and also cannabis. A thorough review of the psychiatric adverse effects of LSD (Abraham & Aldridge 1993) found strong supportive evidence for panic reactions, prolonged schizoaffective psychoses and flashbacks, or more constant 'posthallucinogen perceptual disorder', the latter continuing for as long as five years. Treatments which have occasionally been recommended for perceptual disturbances include haloperidol, simple reassurance and short-term benzodiazepines.

## Steroids

The patterns of anabolic–androgenic steroid use by sports people and body builders, and their physical and psychological side effects and dependence potential, have been reviewed by Korkia (1997) and Beel et al. (1998). Much of the use is by injection, and so many of this population attend needle exchanges, with the advice on reducing infection risks relevant. To increase energy and to go through the 'pain barrier' some will use amphetamines and opiates, either street preparations or illicit pharmaceutical supplies. In the UK the opioid nalbuphine (Nubain) has been abused in this way and, in cases where dependence becomes established, detoxification treatments can be necessary. Some insights into psychological treatment of steroid users have been provided by Corcoran & Longo (1992). In professional sport, screening and testing programmes are required to act as a deterrent to the use of performance-enhancing or illicit drugs, with education and prevention initiatives having a role in many settings (Beel et al. 1998).

## Volatile substances

This is another of the forms of drug misuse which has been studied extensively from a phenomenological point of view, but for which there are no significant treatment avenues. It is known to be hazardous and potentially fatal through several mechanisms, including anoxia and heart arrhythmias (Shepherd 1989), with most deaths in the UK occurring after inhalation of cigarette lighter refills, aerosols and glues. The trends in casualties have shown changes in relation to substances as successive controls have been introduced, rather than overall reductions, indicating the difficulty in addressing the underlying tendency towards adolescent substance misuse. The majority of deaths are consistently in males under 18 years old, with substantial proportions occurring in first-time or near first-time users (Flanagan & Ives 1994). More committed solvent misuse is also problematic in other ways, being strongly linked with conduct disorder and other behavioural problems.

The general management approach to this form of drug misuse is preventive. A small subgroup of users, however, become truly dependent, for instance inhaling glue every 15 minutes of each day for years so that the problem dominates their life, and treatment attempts must be made with such individuals. Some rehabilitation centres will take such cases, and a 'detoxification' may be feasible, usually as an inpatient, with sedative medications used to alleviate distress. Some practical advice for less severe cases has been given by Flanagan & Ives (1994), and the methods of addressing the problem in the UK context have been reviewed by the Advisory Council on the Misuse of Drugs (1995). Specific psychological or psychiatric treatment may be indicated in some cases, including antidepressants.

## Cannabis

There is always plenty of controversy on the subject of cannabis, given that it is probably the least harmful of the drugs currently illegal in the UK and elsewhere. Those favouring decriminalization point out for comparison the hazards of the legally-sanctioned alcohol and tobacco, and claim that the alleged progression on to other drugs would actually be less likely if cannabis did not have to be bought from dealers. They feel it a waste of police time to be occupied with cannabis offences, which make up a huge proportion of total drug offences, and indeed in the UK possession of the drug is increasingly dealt with by caution only. The opposing view is that hazards of present drugs are not a reason to introduce a further one, and that the illegal status presumably acts as some deterrent to more widespread use of a drug which does have significant adverse effects.

In drug services virtually all those dependent on opiates and other more problematic drugs have used cannabis, but that does not answer the question: what proportion of cannabis users make the progression? Kandel & Davies (1992) demonstrated a hierarchy among American adolescents which would apply in many countries: alcohol and tobacco typically preceded the use of cannabis, which in turn preceded the use of hallucinogens and 'pills' and, in a minority, heroin and cocaine. Individuals may stop experimenting at any stage and, with cannabis use arguably becoming more normative, the 'gateway' situation may have moved up a level, with use of hallucinogens and (in the UK) street amphetamine more significant in predicting long-term drug usage. Kandel & Davies (1992) found that early age of first taking cannabis, and heavy use, were associated with subsequent use of heroin and cocaine.

The possible psychological and physical adverse effects of cannabis have been the subject of a recent monograph, and are much debated (Hall et al. 1996, Kalant et al. 1996). The suspicion of an 'amotivational syndrome' has not exactly gone away, but it seems such an entity cannot be distinguished from predominant personality characteristics among cannabis users, and the effects of chronic intoxication (Hall & Solowij 1997). Similarly, heavy cannabis use itself, rather than additional adverse effects, is likely to account for findings of cognitive impairment in long-term users. The evidence for increased risk of psychosis is reasonably strong (Andreasson et al. 1987), but some preexisting vulnerability may be important, as discussed in Chapter 8. Mood disturbances, notably depression and anxiety, may also either reflect an underlying predisposition or the effects of usage, with Troisi et al. (1998) demonstrating a strong relationship between prevalence of psychiatric disorders and extent of cannabis dependence. More direct usage effects are psychomotor impairments, of the kinds which impair driving ability for a period. Respiratory diseases relate to smoking as the method of administration, while there is possibly increased risk of upper digestive tract carcinomas, and adverse fetal effects if cannabis is used in pregnancy.

The extremely high rates of cannabis use among drug misusers generally was demonstrated in a study of amphetamine, cocaine and heroin users in and out of treatment (Robson and Bruce 1997). Of 581 users interviewed, 85% smoked cannabis, three-quarters of those having the drug every day. Budney et al. (1998) found that two-thirds of individuals presenting for treatment of opiate dependence smoked cannabis, nearly all of whom continued to do so during treatment with no apparent adverse effects on outcome. Interestingly, however, the cannabis users appeared to be a generally less stable group, in that they were more likely to report financial difficulties, be involved in drug dealing and engage in sharing needles, as well as being less likely to be married.

As with cigarette smoking, which is discussed below, most individuals attending treatment services do not see cannabis use as something which they definitely want to change, and some see cannabis as highly necessary, for instance in attempts to manage without other drugs or complete a detoxification. Again as with cigarette smoking, however, others may be motivated to reduce cannabis use as part of general behavioural change, and standard drug counselling techniques can be brought to bear. A small minority of cases are referred as primary cannabis users, for instance if their drug use is having adverse social or psychological effects, or when there are occupational implications (Stephens et al. 1993). Here also treatment is in the counselling sphere, unless additional psychiatric medication is required for significant specific conditions.

## Alcohol

Alcohol problems are the subject of many textbooks (e.g. Edwards et al. 1997), and only certain implications which are particularly relevant to the use of alcohol by drug misusers are considered here. The range of psychological adverse effects are well known, commonly including mood disturbances, anxiety as a withdrawal feature and, ultimately, cognitive impairment. Widespread physical effects include detectable liver damage as a relatively early feature in many cases and, although there is much individual variation, liver function tests are a useful indicator of heavy drinking, particularly the gamma glutamyl transferase result. This is reasonably specific to alcohol and also sensitive to decreases or increases in drinking, while increased mean corpuscular volume on a full blood count is a more chronic feature. There are brief questionnaires to identify alcohol problems such as the Alcohol Use Disorders Identification Test (AUDIT) (Babor & Grant 1989), while the classical description of the clinical syndrome of dependence was first delineated in relation to alcohol (Edwards & Gross 1976). This includes the features of increased tolerance to alcohol, withdrawal symptoms and the relief of those symptoms by further drinking, subjective awareness of a compulsion to drink, and the stereotyping of a heavy-drinking routine.

The management of alcohol problems is barely less controversial than that of drug misuse, especially as it has long been recognized that individuals who are given only small amounts of treatment may fare just as well as those who are provided with many successive treatment options (Edwards et al. 1977, Chick et al. 1988). In recent years the limited approach of giving advice on health risks and adhering to recommended safe levels of drinking, plus addressing the most immediate related problems, has been formalized in methods of 'brief intervention' (e.g. Wallace et al. 1988), which are suitable for many people. Beyond that, various forms of counselling are made available, including by Alcoholics Anonymous, whose methods are readily embraced by a subgroup of alcohol misusers. The most useful medications (Chick 1996) are chlordiazepoxide to alleviate alcohol withdrawal symptoms, disulfiram as a deterrent treatment in selected individuals who understand the risk of the potentially fatal disulfiram–ethanol reaction, and acamprosate, a more recently introduced medication which appears to reduce desire for alcohol (Sass et al. 1996). For a substantial minority of severely dependent drinkers detoxification in an inpatient or other residential setting is the only realistic option, and this makes it easier to administer parenteral vitamin B which may be required to reduce the risk of complications such as Korsakoff's psychosis.

Nearly all individuals who present with drug misuse have used alcohol at an earlier stage in their substance-using 'career'. The impression that significant use of alcohol at an early age is associated with various other behavioural and conduct problems and an increased likelihood of subsequent experimentation with drugs has been confirmed in studies (e.g. Federman et al. 1997), the implications therefore being similar to those of early use of cannabis (Kandel & Davies 1992). However, it would seem that as dependence on drugs such as heroin develops, most individuals leave alcohol behind, so that a combined dependence is seen in only a minority of drug misusers in treatment (Gossop et al. 1998). In clinical practice with mainly opiate-dependent individuals there appears to be something of a bimodal distribution, whereby most will have no alcohol at all, a relatively small number will drink in moderation, and some will drink heavily combined with opiates and other drugs, clearly seeking definite intoxication.

This last group can be very difficult to manage, and in particular the standard treatments for alcohol misuse can be compromised by the dual dependence situation. We recognized in Chapter 2 that alcohol is among the substances which some individuals will use to 'boost' the otherwise noneuphoriant effects of methadone, and in cases where drinking is for this purpose the ordinary treatment options for alcohol misuse are perhaps unlikely to be successful. As with individuals who abuse benzodiazepines alongside methadone, there may sometimes be more benefit from altering or adjusting the opioid substitution treatment if adherence to methadone only cannot be achieved. In general, the less obviously that alcohol is used by an individual to fill the euphoria 'gap' left by switching from street heroin to methadone, the more useful direct treatments for alcohol problems may be. In theory, the 12-step methods of Alcoholics Anonymous or Narcotics Anonymous are particularly indicated in those who need to make a commitment to total abstinence from all substances, while we must also recognize that a switch from drugs to alcohol occurs in a proportion of those who attempt drug detoxification (Eklund et al. 1994), especially where detoxification rather than maintenance is an over-ambitious aim.

## Nicotine

In contrast with most of the forms of recreational drug use, cigarette smoking is a type of substance use for which there are reasonably well-established clinical treatments. However, it occupies a peculiar position in relation to our work in drug services in many ways, and not simply because it is legal.

It is sometimes claimed that nicotine is not actually addictive because it does not cause the defining characteristic of intoxication, but such claims come mainly from the tobacco industry, and have been discounted on more general clinical grounds (Stolerman & Jarvis 1995, Hoffman et al. 1996). Craving and the relief of dysphoria in a withdrawal situation are certainly strong, and the high relapse rates are well established. It has been calculated that less than 10% of nearly 20 million people in the USA who stopped smoking for at least one day remained abstinent one year later (Fiore et al. 1994), but a figure in the order of 40% give up eventually, and the vast majority of such individuals do so on their own. Although the equivalent figure of how many people give up heroin on their own is not known, the self-reliance of smokers in this regard is striking when viewed from a drug misuse treatment perspective, and poses questions regarding the requirements for, say, formal relapse prevention in drug misuse. In reality the treatment of the two groups is not often compared, and indeed drug misuse services are notorious for ignoring the whole issue of smoking, even though it is virtually universal among our patients.

Rather than discuss the nuances of the different treatments for smoking cessation, interesting though they are, the most fundamental matter for drug services in this regard is whether to address systematically the matter of smoking at all. It may rightly be said that, on the face of it, most drug misuse patients cannot envisage tackling smoking as well as the drug problem they have actually attended about, although Joseph et al. (1990) found that in a survey of patients admitted for substance misuse treatment, over one-third said they wanted to quit smoking. Furthermore, after that hospital banned smoking on all wards, including those for drug dependency, the proportion rose to 62%, and the new rule was seen as an additional motivating factor. With smoking being legal, the whole area of promoting behaviour change by making regulations for public places is an additional factor which we do not have in drug misuse. Specific addiction counselling methods, however, are routinely deployed in drug misuse clinics, and it may therefore be argued that, far from ignoring smoking, we should be taking the opportunity to assess motivation and offer systematic advice. There is a long way to go, as at present some drug workers will actually offer clients a cigarette as a friendly gesture, and certainly allowing an agitated individual to smoke in a session is fairly routine. Even so, that does not mean that smoking could not be addressed where necessary, and it is likely that drug services will become more involved in this way. Partly, the view of services depends on the model of addiction treatment they apply, as clearly the more socially orientated will not see smoking as having major psychosocial consequences, while a purist model sees more similarities in smoking and drug-taking, as behaviours.

Smoking cessation treatments are a specialized clinical research area, and can be classified as below (Hoffman et al. 1996). Overall, they are considered to approximately double the rates of successful quitting (Hughes 1996).

**Brief therapies**
These are a similar level of treatment to the minimal interventions used by primary care physicians to encourage patients to come off benzodiazepine tranquillizers. Doctors are particularly well placed to advise on smoking cessation, because of the direct health hazards which they can inform patients about. Success rates are reasonable with brief intervention alone (Steele 1995), but results can be improved with additional referral for specialist smoking cessation counselling (Franke et al. 1995).

**Cognitive behaviour therapy**
Some behavioural methods rely on formalization of a basic cutting down, rather than stopping abruptly. Therefore the 'inter-cigarette interval' can

be increased, and amounts smoked at intervals reduced. Cinciripini et al. (1995) achieved one-year abstinence rates of 44% when this approach was combined with intensive counselling. Other methods attempt to weaken the positive reinforcement of smoking by allowing cigarettes at exact times rather than when desired, while relapse prevention methods are used which are similar to those in drug counselling (see Chapter 3). Behaviour therapy may be combined with nicotine replacement treatment, with Hajek (1996) observing that adding nicotine replacement therapy to behaviour therapy leads to large increases in efficacy, while making the addition in treatments the other way round is of uncertain value.

**Nicotine replacement treatment**
Conceptually, this is familiar ground for drug services, as it represents a substitution treatment approach. Nicotine may be administered in a patch, gum, or nasal or oral inhalers, for variable periods. Overall, successful quitting rates appear to be increased by a factor of two to three (Henningfield 1995), with possibly more efficacy in men than women (Perkins 1996). If necessary, use can be prolonged, and may even be on a 'harm-reduction' basis, i.e. to cut down rather than stop – rather as, in practice, some individuals use methadone, or even disulfiram, for respective dependencies.

Saxon et al. (1997) examined transdermal (patch) nicotine replacement therapy specifically in patients admitted for treatment of alcohol or drug misuse. Some 49 individuals elected to try the treatment, representing about a quarter of those offered it, and no psychosocial treatments directed specifically at smoking cessation were used. Patients remained on transdermal nicotine for an average of 19 days, with a desire to return to smoking the main reason for discontinuation. Seven subjects reported tobacco abstinence at 21 days, and five at six weeks, at outpatient follow-up.

In addiction treatment settings which do not currently offer smoking cessation treatment there will be interesting debates as to how appropriate it is to expand into this role. There are other major neglected groups, such as those individuals dependent on prescribed benzodiazepines, and so prioritization and allocation of resources will need critical consideration. In the final analysis, good counselling skills are transferable in addressing the syndrome of dependence, as that applies to the various different substances.

## Summary

Where drug services have a comprehensive responsibility, it is not acceptable to concentrate exclusively on the problems of opiate misusers. It is also not sufficient to apply the basic harm-reduction measures only to nonopiate misusers, with nearly all clinical time spent in managing opiate detoxification or maintenance. Of course there is a tendency for services to be drawn that way, as the problems of addiction are most severe in opiate users and, crucially, there are effective specific clinical treatments in opiate misuse which have no equivalent for most other substances. What must not be lost, however, is skilled drug counselling, of the kind which can sometimes be effective in the absence of any pharmacological interventions. At the time when access to low-threshold methadone treatment was being most emphasized, counselling approaches were neglected, resulting in inadequate responses to other forms of drug misuse.

Even the prioritization of opiate misusers, which in many ways is justifiable because of the severity of problems and the treatments, raises some uncomfortable questions. With other forms of drug misuse commonly precursors to heroin use, do we wait for individuals to become dependent on opiates just so that we can use the treatments which make the most impression? In practice, in many localities it may only be the addiction to opiates which makes users present, but that itself relates to how services are delivered, and if nonopiate users do present we must make our response as effective as possible. Seeing those who have not progressed to heroin could have a vital preventive role, but only if an assertive approach is adopted.

With specific pharmacological treatments extremely limited, the quality of drug counselling is critical in managing nonopiate misuse. Such quality is not easily testable, but there is much available guidance on methods, and supervision plays an important role. Clinical counselling aimed at enabling specific behavioural changes differs markedly from general supportive work, and achieving the right balance is essential if contacts with stimulant users and other groups are to be useful.

Cocaine misuse is one form of nonopiate misuse for which a large number of pharmacological treatments has been tried, which itself suggests that none have been found to be very satisfactory. This is clearly the case, although antidepressants, antipsychotics and tranquillizers may all be indicated in some cases. The general transition in recent years from cocaine hydrochloride to crack has produced higher rates of medical and psychiatric complications, and the levels of usage and adverse effects in individual cases can be extreme. Acute admissions frequently appear necessary, and in cocaine users presenting to services in the UK, inpatient and residential treatment and alternative therapies have been found to be often selected. Behavioural treatments for cocaine misuse include cue exposure and the very different approach of providing material incentives for abstinence, and overall there is clearly no consensus as to the preferable forms of treatment. Some of the same range of treatments have been tried in cocaine-misusing methadone patients, with similarly limited success, and in such patients various alterations in the opioid management approach may be more effective.

Amphetamine misusers are an unduly neglected group, considering the prevalence of usage, the links with subsequent heroin use, and the rates of HIV-risk behaviours and psychiatric complications. A policy of amphetamine prescribing is sometimes looked to in order to attract users into treatment, but this is only suitable for a very small minority. There are no other specific treatments, and counselling approaches must be substantially relied upon. Many amphetamine users who are seen in clinics have ongoing fluctuating psychotic symptoms, and skilled psychiatric management is required. Ecstasy users are similarly mainly seen when psychiatric adverse effects develop, which are of uncertain causation, as are the sometimes fatal physical complications.

Benzodiazepine misuse, as opposed to licit ordinary-dose benzodiazepine dependence, is usually a secondary form of drug misuse. The combination with opiates is the most commonly seen in clinics and, as with secondary cocaine misuse, manipulation of the opioid treatment may be required. Controlled benzodiazepine prescribing is indicated in some situations, especially detoxification from high-dose misuse. In our area another pharmaceutical drug which patients will combine with methadone is cyclizine, which produces bizarre psychological disturbances and other characteristic problems, but for which there is no direct treatment.

The adverse effects of cannabis, beyond direct effects of usage such as psychomotor impairment and mood disturbances, are much debated but probably include psychotic features in predisposed individuals. The problems of alcohol misuse are well known, and the available treatments can be employed in the minority of drug misusers who have a combined dependence, although other strategies are often required. Use of alcohol or cannabis at a young age is an indication of other psychological and behavioural problems, of the kind commonly associated with volatile substance misuse. This and steroid use have predominantly physical direct complications, and such users are rarely encountered in clinical drug services.

Those two observations apply even more to cigarette smokers, and drug services are criticized for largely ignoring smoking in their own patients. As public pressure to cut smoking steps up all the time, involvement with this group is likely to be increasingly advised, and there are some reasonably well-established treatments. Drug counselling skills should be transferable to this group, but only where a systematic clinical approach is adopted.

# Part II

# Providing clinical services

# 5

## Community drug services

### Introduction

This book is written from the perspective of working within multidisciplinary community-based treatment services for drug misusers. In the UK these are not a minority type of service subsumed under more institutionalized treatment, but rather they represent the main model of treatment delivery in this specialty in most areas. They are primarily clinical, with most of the work comprising counselling of various kinds for the drug misusers who have been referred, along with medical input and the provision of pharmacological treatments. The teams are part of the National Health Service, with funding usually coming jointly from health and social services. Typically most workers are community psychiatric nurses or social workers, with much overlap in the type of casework undertaken. The extent to which teams are involved in nonclinical projects, such as needle exchange schemes, outreach, drug information or relatives' groups, depends largely on the availability of other services, particularly from the nonstatutory sector, and carving out a suitable role for a clinical community drug service is an important challenge. Many lessons have been learnt as such services have emerged from the shadow of the previously dominant drug dependence units (DDUs), as a brief history of this process of development will illustrate.

### Historical development

The formation of nonmedical multidisciplinary community drug teams (CDTs) was recommended in a highly influential report of the Advisory Council on the Misuse of Drugs, the UK's central advisory body which is set up by statute (Advisory Council on the Misuse of Drugs 1982). Among a series of reports, this one laid down the desirable structure of treatment and rehabilitation services for drug misusers within the country, and it was envisaged that each health district, with populations of around a quarter of a million people, would have such a drug team. Their main role was seen not so much as direct provision of clinical treatment to limited numbers of users, but the facilitation of treatment and rehabilitation by a wider network of professionals. This nonmedical team would therefore have links with a local consultant psychiatrist in drug misuse and their junior doctors, and primary care physicians, as well as with nonstatutory drug agencies, probation, social services and other organizations in contact with drug users. The CDT had premises in a community location, preferably in a town centre, and joint treatment for a client would usually comprise counselling at the CDT base plus appointments at the local consultant's outpatient clinic, or their own primary care physician's office. Over and above these local clinical services each of the regions, which could comprise 10–20 health districts, would have a more specialized drug misuse service with full-time consultants, bigger medical and multidisciplinary teams and additional facilities such as an inpatient unit. Such services were expected to generally treat the more difficult cases, and were typically based where there had previously been the substantial DDUs.

These Advisory Council on the Misuse of Drugs recommendations can be seen as very formative in the deinstitutionalization of drug misuse treatment in the UK, as previously the DDUs had overseen the treatment of most of the known addicts in their areas, with the disadvantages of long distance travelling for patients and lack of involvement of generic services. As rates of drug misuse generally increased, with clinical treatments clearly indicated for a substantial proportion of the new heroin users, it was recognized that general practitioners and a wide range of other doctors and associated clinicians would need to be involved. These principles were reinforced still further a few years later as drug misusers became implicated in the HIV epidemic, when there was a consequent emphasis on widespread low-threshold treatment (Advisory Council on the Misuse of Drugs 1988, 1989). Throughout the 1980s many posts were therefore created to form the new CDTs, who were required to have a role in training as well as the provision and facilitation of treatment.

The model of community drug services has endured, with important changes of emphasis which are detailed below. As time has progressed they have become even more the focus of treatment for most areas, since changes in the National Health Service have meant that the conventional regional and district structure in administration and provision has largely been dismantled. With decentralization and some scaling down of regional services, most districts covering populations of a quarter to half a million are needing to become more self-sufficient in drug misuse treatment. The largest services which previously operated on a regional basis

Table 5.1. *The work of community drug teams*

====

*Composition of teams*
Community psychiatric nurses, social workers, other drug counsellors,
management, administration, plus medical input

*Catchment area*
Local, defined

*Clinical treatment*
Triage
Facilitation of treatment by others
Direct treatment of medium-severity cases

*General roles*
Counselling
Advice and information
Telephone help-line
Drop-in service
Needle exchange
Outreach
General medical services

====

Based on Strang et al. (1992)

are needing to reevaluate their role, concentrating for instance on the
newer methods of inpatient opiate detoxification or on providing outpatient prescribing services for individuals who require nonstandard
medication regimes.

We will focus here on treatment within community drug services, as
these have evolved in the face of changing demands.

## Changes in emphasis

The practicalities of working in CDTs, as services stood at the start of the
1990s, were described by Strang et al. (1992). The main aspects are
summarized in Table 5.1.

The multidisciplinary composition of teams was seen as fundamental
to this service model. Strang et al. (1992) noted that this related strongly
to the liaison element of the work so that, for instance, links with social
services would be more effectively forged if the approach came from a
social worker in a CDT. As CDTs took on more direct treatment the

benefits had more to do with skill mix for their own clinical work, and were perhaps more arguable. Most posts were for community psychiatric nurses and social workers, with some unqualified drug workers who might be ex-users. Having workers from different disciplines with their own 'line managers' could pose problems for overall team management, and often there was a coordinator post to include that role.

A complement of four full-time and two part-time workers, including a secretary and a coordinator, was considered about average at that time. The catchment area would be absolutely defined, with the advantage that the team would get to know their local area and its services well, and make the links with other agencies in the community. As in other specialties in psychiatry, the community ethos of treatment relates to links of this kind, as well as to location of services and an emphasis on visits to home and other settings.

Initially, medical treatment was seen as an aspect which was provided elsewhere, through liaison as indicated above. Gradually the nonmedical and medical elements of treatment have become more integrated, to the extent that the term 'CDT' is somewhat outdated as describing nonmedical personnel only. Partly this integration has been desired, with consultants for instance preferring to do their clinics for drug misusers at CDT premises, rather than have patients brought to them by workers. As well as the benefits of convenience for the patient and better communication between doctor and team, this gets away from the perception of a worker acting as a separate advocate for a drug user in their dealings with the doctor. Also, however, prescribing in particular has had to move 'in-house' as drug services acknowledged that they needed to carry out direct treatment in a large proportion of cases. The original CDT concept implied a kind of 'triage' system, in which drug users with routine prescription needs could be treated by their own primary care physicians with guidance, some especially problematic individuals might need referral to a regional centre, and only a limited number would require all aspects of management to be from the drug service. Assessing nearly a decade of the setting-up and operating of CDTs, Strang et al. (1992) observed that '[because] the extent of collaboration from generic colleagues (especially general practitioners) has been poor ... an unplanned abandonment of the original consultancy role for the CDT is widely evident, as CDT workers have become more actively involved in the delivery of care'. Offering in-house prescribing might be considered to compound the difficulty of encouraging generic services to become involved with treating drug misusers, but it has been a necessary pragmatic development. At a time when the importance of contact with services was being emphasized because of HIV, drug teams with medical services were found to see six times as many heroin users, three times as many amphetamine users, and five times as many injecting drug misusers overall, than comparable teams without such input (Strang et al. 1991).

In mentioning the possible general roles for a CDT as listed in Table 5.1, Strang et al. (1992) suggest that all except drug counselling and the provision of advice and information lie outside the original brief (Advisory Council on the Misuse of Drugs 1982). Drug counselling is of course central to the work of nonmedical members of drug treatment services, and is considered further below. Services will inevitably feel the need to give advice to drug users and relatives contacting them in their area, but use can also be made of the various national telephone helplines and drugs information outlets. The division of activities between a clinical service and any local 'street agencies' run by nonstatutory organizations for drug users is important to establish, and the latter may for instance provide leaflets, information and contact telephone numbers on a drop-in basis. There are inevitable areas of overlap, but it is generally more appropriate for informal contacts, nonspecific support and needle exchange to also be at the street agency. The difficulties of reconciling injecting equipment provision with clinical sessions, in which some users may not fully acknowledge their additional drug use, have been recognized ever since harm-reduction measures were introduced, and even where both kinds of assistance are provided from the same service there needs to be a degree of separation.

Outreach services in drug misuse (Grund et al. 1992) may include distributing injecting equipment, informal health promotion, efforts to recruit younger heroin users into treatment, or initiatives related to other drugs, such as advising on safer use of stimulants in nightclub attenders. Once again, in areas where there is a street drug agency this work is increasingly seen as being mainly in their province, for a number of reasons. Some of these are practical, relating to unusual working hours and conditions, while others are to do with the various skills required for different kinds of work, and the need to orientate professional staff more to clinical treatment. In the current employment and medico-legal climates there are potential problems in having health service staff involved in the more inventive fringes of drug outreach work, just as there are pitfalls the other way round in, for instance, having ex-users advising on prescribed treatments.

There are precedents for both statutory and nonstatutory services offering general health care sessions for drug misusers who do not contact general practitioners. Morrison & Ruben (1995) described such a scheme, in which a general practitioner provided four sessions a week at a centre aimed at HIV-preventive activities. The authors pointed out that not only did many drug users fail to access direct treatment for drug misuse or ordinary primary health care services from primary care physicians, but many more were not even registered with a doctor. Their service was also aimed at prostitutes, and concentrated on HIV and hepatitis testing, hepatitis B vaccination, sexually transmitted infection screening, and contraception. It has long been recognized that drug services tend not to be active enough in pursuing hepatitis B vaccination (Farrell et al. 1990), with a study of drug misusers in police custody finding that only 10% were aware of its availability, despite nearly 50% being in contact with treatment services (Payne-James et al. 1994).

Some further effective elements of community drug service provision, and also some of the related problems, can be illustrated by brief discussion of our own services.

## Local provision

### Community Health Sheffield Substance Misuse Service

Sheffield is a particularly difficult place to establish treatment services, largely due to two historical legacies. In the mid-1980s the prescribing clinic was disbanded and virtually replaced by a policy of short-term detoxification and referral to Phoenix House in the city, a phenomenon actually known as the 'Sheffield effect' (Liappas et al. 1987, Preston 1996c). Many of those who were obvious maintenance candidates sought treatment in neighbouring towns, typically at clinics where they knew they could obtain high-dose, injectable or combination prescriptions. Those individuals are gradually returning and are presenting, along with all the new cases, to a clinic which, because of the previous approach, has a small capacity. Also, in terms of community treatment, an ideological over-investment in the collective model of having statutory and non-statutory workers carrying out essentially the same duties in one team, has had various adverse consequences. The most problematic of these were inappropriate roles for the workers with different backgrounds, a lack of clarity regarding clinical counselling rather than nonspecific supportive work, and a curious imbalance whereby community psychiatric nurses in the collective team would be drawn into the role of advocate for a user when dealing with treatment services, including those containing their own clinical colleagues. Overall, the provision for treatment posts rather than other initiatives has traditionally been very limited, and so we are having to build a service up from a low point.

Sheffield is a city of approximately 600 000 population, best known for its steel-making industry. With manufacturing generally in decline, there has been the usual growth in industries such as retail and leisure, but there is also high unemployment. In terms of drug misuse, Sheffield is fairly representative of the UK's other major cities, with heroin, cocaine, amphetamine and the other illicit drugs all widely used. As well as the city's own drug misusers, there is a significant additional population comprising those who stay here after dropping out of residential rehabilitation at Phoenix House, having initially come to Sheffield from elsewhere.

In 1995 the clinical team came together as a service, some posts having previously been located within the nonstatutory agency, as indicated. We work from part of a large health service premises in the city centre, convenient for public transport. Although not an absolute requirement, the preference at present is for referrals to come from a user's primary care physician, which is for several reasons. We will require that patients have a primary care physician for general medical care and so this confirmation is useful. Also, we will look to develop shared care where possible, while there is as well an acknowledged gate-keeping function, in that we would simply not be able to cater for self-referrals or even the numbers who present at drop-in services. It may also be claimed that a user having seen a primary care physician to request a referral to us shows some motivation, but in reality this is not a simple association. From a starting point of staffing much below recommended levels, future initiatives will need to be costed developments, such as a forthcoming plan for referrals to be accepted direct from the probation service in a court diversion scheme.

The service is for both drug and alcohol misusers, but relatively we treat a higher proportion of drug cases, with alcohol misusers being also substantially managed within general psychiatry. The medical, social work, psychology and service manager posts cover both patient groups, but there are separate community psychiatric nurse posts for each specialism. In drug misuse two community psychiatric nurses work with the general caseload, with additional posts specifically for primary care liaison and for short-term community detoxification cases. Some of our posts are part-time, while there are additional staff for the prescribing clinic and the five inpatient beds which we have at one of the psychiatric hospitals.

We receive around 25 referrals a week, and these are allocated to workers at a weekly clinical meeting, as in many other services. Many nonmedical appointments are by way of home visits, while we also use our base for appointments and clinics, but not for methadone dispensing, because of regulations relating to the premises. At present, all dispensing for outpatient treatment is at the community pharmacies selected by each user, although that policy may have to be changed as it is relatively expensive. Many patients have both nonmedical and medical workers involved but, as has already been explained, that is not always necessary or feasible. Several more specific aspects of the deployment of this service are described in the relevant sections of the book.

The main street drug agency in the city, the Rockingham Drug Project, provides services including needle exchange, support on a drop-in basis, information, outreach, acupuncture, and a separate young drug users' project. The Phoenix House organization now also employs community drug workers, and there are several other nonclinical helping organizations for drug misusers. Once again, ideally, there would be more direct referral routes from these agencies to a clinical service, but there has not so far been the scope for this. Because of the numbers of drug misusers involved there clearly needs to be a big expansion in treatment provision, the question being what kind of services would best fulfil the city's needs. It is likely that our service will operate partly as a tertiary service, while also specializing in detoxification treatments for early-stage users and the mangement of special groups such as pregnant users and dual diagnosis cases, with the more routine methadone treatment provided by a secondary service operated by primary care physicians. The latter model of development is discussed in Chapter 6.

### North Nottinghamshire Community Drug Service
The staff complement for this team is more realistic for the area covered and so, whereas in Sheffield we have had a major development challenge, here there are more established aspects of the work which can be considered features of a model community drug service.

The North Nottinghamshire service covers a population of 420 000 spread over a wide geographical area. There are no large city conurbations, the largest town in the area, Mansfield, having a population of 70 000. Mining and other traditional industries are again in decline, with high unemployment in some of the towns but also some more prosperous areas. The drug scene is influenced by those of the nearest cities, Nottingham and Sheffield, but some features are absent, so that for instance there is little use of crack cocaine. Heroin has become easily available throughout this area in the past few years, but before that the towns were strongly characterized by amphetamine use, and this is still very prevalent.

The service has its base in a converted brewery premises in Mansfield town centre. It is the only drug service in the area and so, more than in Sheffield, it takes on some of the roles which would otherwise be in the province of a nonstatutory agency. Staffing comprises the clinical manager, three community psychiatric nurses, one social worker, two drug counsellors, two drug workers for young people, and two criminal justice system workers. Having separate workers for young people (mainly under 18 years old) is considered important because of the substantially different emphasis in the work, which includes outreach, help with aspects such as accommodation, education or employment, liaison with youth workers, and introducing users to harm-reduction and the idea of treatment services. The criminal justice system workers operate closely with the courts, facilitating treatment where appropriate for drug-using offenders. The main needle exchange is also within the premises, although entirely self-contained and with separate workers. There are also close links with the health promotion service in the same building.

The only medical input within the service consists of two sessions a week from myself, and one session from a local primary care physician. We do two clinics per week, in which we provide the pharmacological treatments for patients whose management plan has been formulated by their keyworker. In my own sessions there may also be psychiatric assessments, typically in stimulant misusers or those with significant dual diagnosis problems. This responsive way of working, rather than operating a system where patients are put forward for decisions to be taken mainly by the doctor, places much of the responsibility for selecting appropriate treatments on the drug workers, and high standards are inevitably required. A combination throughout the team of a generally patient-friendly but assertive clinical approach, good supervision, and realistic (although still very demanding!) caseloads means that the system works well, and it is extremely rare for a doctor to go against the treatment plan made by the drug worker.

The limitation in medical sessions in the service also has wider effects on the general balance of treatment provision. Because of the strong counselling emphasis, relatively few users present of the kind who are exclusively motivated to manipulate supplies of medication to misuse, with no associated treatment inclination. There is a related potential risk that those who require maintenance methadone but are simply 'not psychologically-minded' may also be deterred, but the team have the skills to separate the two groups, and such individuals are definitely accommodated. A more direct effect is that local primary care physicians simply cannot have the expectation that all pharmacological treatment of drug misusers can be provided by the drug service, and through good liaison the level of involvement of primary care physicians in prescribing recommended treatments is high.

There are various operational aspects of the North Nottinghamshire service which work particularly well in practice, as follows:

- Sectorization
  Each of the workers within the core team primarily covers one geographical sector, based on local government boundaries. The advantages of sectorization are well recognized, and include not only the worker becoming familiar with local services, personnel and drug scenes, but also the local users getting to know the worker. Often referrals are enabled in this way, and sometimes the worker will already know of a newly presenting individual through other contacts, which helps in general assessment. There is also a back-up system, in which one other worker takes a proportion of referrals from the area and makes the contacts to a lesser degree, which is useful at times such as holiday cover or periods when additional input is required.
- Any referral source, including self-referral
  In this service referrals can be taken from any source, including primary care, probation, social services or other agencies, or individuals may self-refer. Self-referral is actually the most frequent route, which is probably a good indicator of the general level of satisfaction with the service. This wider policy, as opposed to our practice in Sheffield of accepting mainly from primary care physicians and having no self-presentations, is made possible by the higher staffing level and an absence of a large city concentration of opiate users – the number of referrals received weekly in the two services is remarkably similar.
- Duty worker system
  Each weekday afternoon one of the workers is available to see self-referrals or other individuals presenting, and to give telephone advice to anyone who requires it. Such contacts need to be reasonably brief and, in the case of new referrals, usually initial details are taken so that a worker can be allocated to the individual at the weekly team meeting. In some situations where an urgent response is indicated, such as

starting naltrexone in an individual presenting drug-free (see Chapter 3), this is arranged after appropriate testing. Relevant preliminary advice is given in all newly-presenting cases, including written information where possible. For other contacts, the drug worker system is designed to reduce the frustration for individuals of having nobody available to answer queries, including when a client's own worker may be out doing community visits.

- Emphasis on home and community visits
  With a large geographical area it is considered unreasonable to expect clients to usually attend the Mansfield base. They need to do so for the set medical clinic sessions, but the vast majority of appointments with the drug workers are either at home or at other community offices. Once again the advantages of home visits are well known, including seeing a clients's circumstances and talking to relatives or partners, while we also do not expect individuals undergoing quick detoxifications to travel. The sectorization of the service makes for increased efficiency of a community policy, in terms of travelling time and costs.
- Active key working
  The key worker role is considered very important with all clients of the service. Once a worker is allocated to a case, they take all of the main treatment decisions, with supervision provided. In normal circumstances such decisions should not be over-ridden either in duty worker contacts or by the prescribing doctor, and clients are made aware of this. Because the system is adhered to consistently there are relatively few attempts to manipulate the service, and in general this approach is well accepted.

  The key worker role is a very active one with, for instance, much support and encouragement provided to young users who wish to detoxify. In established methadone maintenance patients, medical appointments may occur only two to three times per year, with all the intervening contacts with the key worker. Here the agenda is not to apply inappropriate pressure to detoxify, but to assist and advise regarding various important additional aspects, ranging from social problems to engagement with general medical care. In all clients for whom treatment is underway or planned, regular contact is strongly encouraged.

Much of the work of this service and other community drug services comes into the category of drug counselling, and this will now be examined in a little more detail.

## Drug counselling

This term potentially includes a wide range of approaches, from informal support to specific techniques such as motivational interviewing (Noonan & Moyers 1997), and the particular methods adopted in rehabilitation centres or 12-step programmes. In clinical services in the UK and elsewhere, a concept of drug counselling is prevalent which includes providing various types of practical advice in different situations, but also incorporates elements which are relatively targeted in aiming at behavioural change; in Chapter 3 we discussed such approaches in relation to detoxification and relapse prevention. This kind of work is fundamental to drug services as, to varying degrees, counselling is indicated for virtually all individuals who present. Table 5.2 indicates some of the main elements of drug counselling, which are not highly specialized in nature, but may be useful measures to adopt with or without the application of more specific clinical treatments. Particularly in forms of drug misuse for which no pharmacological treatments are indicated, such approaches may be the most useful input in helping an individual reduce harmful behaviours and cut down or stop drug-taking.

Harm reduction is in itself a large subject, but the particular measures which should be adopted by each individual can readily be covered in counselling. Sexual risk-taking behaviour is notoriously more difficult to change than behaviours relating to drugs, and both aspects must be addressed. Health advice may be concerned with specific adverse effects of drugs, side-effects of medication, general aspects such as nutrition, or testing and vaccination for infectious complications. Beyond basic harm-reduction advice, individuals can be counselled more specifically regarding tactics for reducing drug usage, changing route, and modifying drug-taking in various ways. There may be related lifestyle changes to consider, to do with networks of friends, social activities, or more major changes such as moving area. Dealing with cravings overlaps with this, but involves other aspects such as various distraction techniques.

There are further areas in which the counselling becomes somewhat more specialized, and psychological, in nature, relating to difficulties which are common in drug misusers. It may be necessary to advise on methods of coping with stress, to enhance problem-solving or social skills, or to address significant problems of low self-esteem, anxiety or depression. With the casework of drug team members generally being very similar this may fall to most types of worker, but clearly community psychiatric nurses and psychologists are particularly well placed to admin-

Table 5.2. *Elements of general drug counselling*

| |
|---|
| Harm-reduction advice – drugs, sex |
| Health advice |
| Changing drug-taking behaviours |
| Changing lifestyle |
| Dealing with cravings, stress |
| Problem solving |
| Social skills |
| Psychological aspects – self-esteem, anxiety and depression |

ister counselling of this kind. The management of drug users with definite additional psychiatric disorders is considered further in Chapter 8.

## Summary

Most drug misusers in treatment in the UK are managed by community services. The major development of these services took place in the 1980s, following an advisory recommendation that each health district should have a multidisciplinary community drug team (CDT). The expansion of services gained further momentum as more treatment was encouraged when drug misusers were implicated in the HIV epidemic. The original intention was that the CDT's main role would be the facilitation of treatment by others but, probably inevitably, they have been required to undertake substantially direct treatment themselves. There has been criticism of the lack of enthusiasm for drug misuse treatment outside the specialized services while, paradoxically, the very presence of services to some extent deters this.

CDTs were intended to be multidisciplinary, which has remained an enduring principle throughout subsequent development. Much of the clinical work involved counselling of various kinds, with pharmacological treatments provided by the local psychiatrist specializing in drug misuse, or clients' own primary care physicians. Gradually, medical input has tended to become more integrated with the multidisciplinary service, with the availability of at least some 'in-house' prescribing considered desirable. Services have also been required to become more self-sufficient, not only because of the uncertainty of generic involvement, but because changes in the National Health Service have led to some dismantling of the originally recommended structure of which CDTs were one part. At the outset there were links with larger regional services for drug misusers, which would accept particularly problematic cases, but this is now not always so, and community drug services, as they have evolved, need to be able to cater for most clinical situations.

The provision of nonclinical services such as needle exchange, general advice and information, support on a drop-in basis, and outreach initiatives, is probably best undertaken by a nonstatutory street drug agency, where available. Some of this work differs significantly in nature from the core work of clinical services, although there needs to be overlap in localities where there are not both types of agency present. It is important that there is adequate distinction between nonspecific supportive work and advocacy on the one hand, and more systematic clinically-based interventions and prescribing on the other, otherwise problematic issues can be raised for both users and staff. In a clinical service an assertive approach is often necessary, with much skill required to combine this with patient friendliness. Organizational aspects are important in making a community service responsive, efficient and effective.

Systematic drug counselling should be available for all clients of community drug services, and often forms a major part of treatment. Various specific elements of counselling may be indicated according to individual needs, across the range of differing situations and types of drug misuse.

# 6

## Treatment of drug misuse in primary care

### Introduction

The treatment of drug misusers in primary care is a controversial subject which arouses particularly strong feelings. Although there are many examples of entirely satisfactory treatment and of impressive schemes run by primary care physicians, the problems of managing this group in the primary care setting are also frequently highlighted. Around the time I came to Sheffield, the leading article in a primary care newsletter exhorted physicians to 'man the barricades' against involvement in treating drug misusers, which was a reaction to a previous over-optimistic plan for most drug misuse treatment to take place routinely in that setting. There is certainly no room for naivety in considering drug misuse and primary care, as the primary care situation is especially vulnerable to exploitation by such patients, and most physicians know this very well.

In planning services there must be recognition of both the problems and the advantages of treatment in primary care, and we will discuss these here. There is wide variation in the extent to which primary care physicians become engaged in managing drug misusers, and this will be examined in relation to attitudes, training and other aspects. The chapter mainly adopts the perspective of treatment in the UK, where there are no major restrictions on managing drug misusers in primary care, and therefore there is substantial experience to draw on.

### Problems

The particular problems of treatment in primary care are identified first, as these strongly influence attitudes and approaches to treatment. The ones which appear most important in the UK treatment system are indicated in Table 6.1.

Although many drug misusers undoubtedly keep a low profile, particularly if no direct treatment is being offered, high rates of usage of primary

Table 6.1. *Particular problems of managing drug misusers in primary care*

Tend to be time-consuming patients
Opportunistic contacts relatively easy
Difficult to establish reliability of information
Setting not suited to managing incidents
If treatment offered, demand may be excessive

care services are also often found. Leaver et al. (1992) showed that intravenous heroin users had more routine and emergency appointments than control subjects, failed to attend arranged appointments more often, and received more medication even when methadone was excluded from analysis. In a survey in London 92% of responding primary care physicians were of the opinion that drug misusers take up more consultation time than other patients (Deehan et al. 1997), while HIV-positive status has also been found to increase contact (Ronald et al. 1992). Time is particularly an issue in primary care, where appointments are short, and the temptation to curtail an appointment by issuing a prescription as the route of least resistance is well recognized.

Drug misusers often attend with that aim in mind, and such opportunistic presentations are easier in primary care than in a clinic setting. In clinics we may simply decline to see a methadone patient who is requesting extra medication between appointments, but the UK general practice system is such that contact is harder to prohibit. There may be particular difficulties in corroborating a history of drug misuse in newly-presenting individuals, or claims made by ongoing patients, again with time an important factor. Adherence to contracts and urine monitoring may be undermined if it is feared that insistence may provoke an incident or aggressive outburst, which are difficult to contain in this setting. Finally, since many primary care physicians do not treat drug misusers, those who offer methadone in particular are likely to encounter an undue demand. In Glasgow it was estimated that there was a ratio of 20 injecting drug users to every primary care physician (Ralston & Kidd 1996), but clearly treatment is not distributed like that, and anyway individuals may present as temporary patients.

Greenwood (1992) identified broader factors which operate as obstacles to drug misuse treatment in primary care, which were addressed in the subsequent highly successful involvement of physicians in treatment in Edinburgh. They included lack of familiarity with drug use and

---

Box 6.1. *Levels of interest of primary care physicians in treating drug misusers*

*Level 1*
Substantially involved, e.g. working in a drug misuse service or providing special clinics in primary care. Particularly interested in this patient group.

*Level 2*
More limited involvement, e.g. offering treatment to a small number in conjunction with a drug service. No major objections, provided situation can be contained.

*Level 3*
Not currently offering treatment but would do so if additional training and support were made available.

*Level 4*
Opposed to treatment taking place in primary care, perhaps vehemently. Probably also reluctant to have drug misusers as patients for general medical care. May be a personal opinion or a practice policy.

---

drug users, personal reactions to the condition, anxieties about treatments, disillusionment at relapse rates, and basic matters such as fear of violence and financial implications of treatment.

## Levels of interest

Box 6.1 illustrates four characteristic levels at which primary care physicians are involved in treating drug misusers. It refers primarily to the direct treatment of drug misuse itself rather than providing general medical services, and to systematic treatment rather than aspects such as one-off prescriptions.

Clearly the extent of involvement with this patient group relates to personal interest, training, practice-wide policies, and a range of attitudes towards drug misuse treatment which have been the subject of many surveys (Glanz 1986, Abed & Neira-Munoz 1990, Ralston & Kidd 1996, Deehan et al. 1997, Davies & Huxley 1997). Indeed, in the UK the usefulness of further surveys of attitudes would appear to be limited, with already many consistent findings, and differences which are likely to be largely due to methodological aspects or features of local service provision. The most consistently reported views are broadly that drug misusers are relatively difficult to manage, training is lacking, and liaison with specialist services is generally desired, and these are reflected in studies in other countries (e.g. Vader & Aufseesser 1993, Duszynski et al. 1995, Chowdhury & Bhattacharjee 1995). Several studies find that younger physicians are likely to have more positive attitudes and more involvement with drug misusers, no doubt partly due to increased training and general familiarity with the subject.

Training in drug misuse for primary care physicians can be seen as inherently beneficial across all levels of involvement. It has rarely been adequate at medical school or even in vocational training schemes, and further targeted instruction, made relevant to the patient groups which are encountered, is generally appreciated. In terms of the schema in Box 6.1, the best use of limited training time is not so much to attempt drugs awareness work with those primary care physicians in level 4, but rather to prioritize input for those who have an inclination to be involved in treatment. In many places there is an agenda of recruiting more physicians into overall treatment provision, in which case those in level 3 can be seen as a suitable target group for training, while doctors in level 2 may more value the direct clinical liaison.

The recent survey by Deehan et al. (1997), however, suggests that the role of training may not be as critical or as fruitful as has often been assumed. With just over half of primary care physicians in an outer London area responding, only a minority considered that more training or support from local services would encourage them to work with drug misusers, whereas the position was reversed for alcohol misusers. Special payments would apparently also not help and, bearing in mind that the nonrespondents were older and likely to be even less inclined to treatment, the authors conclude bluntly that 'we find a GP workforce who are only minimally involved with this group, do not wish to be involved with this work, do not consider it appropriate for the primary care setting, and would not be greatly influenced in these matters by the provision of additional training, support, or incentives'. Even in the study by Davies & Huxley (1997), which presents itself as much more optimistic, the largest proportion of physicians considered that the treatment of opiate users was beyond their competence, and that they should refer all on to a specialist service.

The importance of the limited overall enthusiasm of primary care physicians for managing drug misusers lies not in any kind of competition between specialist services and primary care, as manifestly there are more than enough drug misusers to go round, and an integrated approach with different options would seem highly desirable. The problem is rather that the physicians' involvement is far short of that which is repeatedly recommended by advisory bodies (Advisory Council on the Misuse of Drugs 1988, Department of Health 1991, Duszynski et al. 1995) and, given the increasing pressures on primary care from all sides, it would appear that policy makers must become more realistic in their expectations of levels of treatment. One additional aspect is relevant which barely features in the surveys, namely that with most practices being partnerships, it is common for some doctors who would be amenable to doing drug misuse treatment to be over-ridden by a general practice policy.

## Positive treatment approaches

The features of the primary care setting which place it at an advantage in the general management of drug misusers have been reviewed from the perspective of the UK (Robertson 1989) and the USA (Haverkos & Stein 1995). In many areas drug misuse is one of the most common health problems in young people, and physicians may have early indications of this in individuals, through family and other contacts. Drug users may be seen early in their careers, or in the development of heroin dependence following recreational drug use, and opportunities can be taken to intervene with treatments such as lofexidine detoxification before the problem worsens or there are delays with other services. A holistic approach can readily encompass health education, screening, contraceptive advice and hepatitis B screening, while in terms of regulations, virtually any of the direct treatments for drug misuse may be provided. Because of the problems, however, there is much interest in primary care treatment either being supported by the specialist service or forming part of an organized scheme, and these models will be considered.

### Liaison
Most clinical drug misuse services in the UK devote some of their time to providing counselling and other support for patients who are being prescribed for by primary care physicians. This model of working tends to be very well received, as typically there are benefits to all parties. The prescriber feels less isolated and can be assured that more specialized counselling and monitoring are occurring, while the drug service not only spreads the burden of prescribing but has access to more information and links within patients' own communities. In this situation a drug misuser's

Table 6.2. *Roles of a primary care liaison drug worker*

| |
|---|
| Advise on pharmacological treatments, including detoxification packages |
| Counselling and monitoring of patients prescribed for by primary care physicians |
| Facilitate transfer between primary and secondary services |
| Training of primary health care teams |
| Liaison with related community services |

appointments may be able to be at home or at the consulting room rather than at the drug treatment centre, still with a specialized treatment approach. A service may have one or more identified practice liaison workers or, alternatively, all team members may undertake this work with physicians in their area. Given that the role involves advising doctors on the use of various medications, such workers should usually have a clinical background, and in practice most are community psychiatric nurses. A practical account of the work has been given by King (1997) and the elements which we find to be most important are indicated in Table 6.2.

In Sheffield we have separate general practice liaison posts, while in North Nottinghamshire each of the community team members undertakes this work according to geographical area; either system can be satisfactory. The main part of the role is clinical work with patients of primary care physicians, including counselling which is arranged at whichever location suits the patients, and ensuring that urine monitoring takes place. The worker is involved in specifying contracts for treatment, and should advise on the exact use of pharmacological treatments. The protocols for detoxification with lofexidine and other medications are those outlined in Appendix 1 and, both in the case of those and ongoing methadone, we find it best to agree exactly what a patient will receive, so that the physician is not pressurized for extra medication. Once again this aspect is usually welcomed by the doctors, and it is made clear that any representations about changing a treatment plan should be made to the drug worker. Apart from the direct clinical role, such a worker should be a point of contact regarding referrals to the secondary service, or situations in which a physician can transfer a patient back the other way. They are well placed to play a main part in training, not only with physicians but with the full primary health care team, and links can also be made with any relevant community services, such as social services, probation or support organizations. In areas where there is an established secondary service, the model of liaison work is the main method of enhancing primary care physician involvement with drug misusers. Given a suitably reliable and clinical approach on the part of workers, the model undoubtedly works very well, and many developments of this kind are currently taking place.

### Primary care physician secondary services

This is another emerging model, in which secondary treatment is carried out not by drug misuse specialists as such, but by physicians with additional expertise and training in the subject. Sometimes such schemes have arisen as the main service in areas where there has not been substantial provision from psychiatric services, but there is no reason why both should not coexist, provided there is not undue competition for very limited resources. What does need to be acknowledged is that such schemes effectively represent an admission that it is unrealistic, and probably inappropriate, that each drug misuser be managed by his or her own physician, and planners must be aware of the reasons, as noted above. It could be claimed that if patients are to have a secondary service, then it should be a fully specialized one, but it may be that primary care physician schemes can form better links with outright primary care and be more suitable for some types of patients. Patients who are stabilized on ongoing methadone and who are making unproblematic progress are one group who, it is often recommended, are transferred from specialist services to primary care; in Sheffield we find that the most efficient arrangement is to manage large numbers of such cases within a newly developed practitioner-led secondary service, while utilizing outright primary care mainly for more time-limited treatments, when the physicians are agreeable. Successful transfer of stabilized methadone maintenance patients to an intermediate level of support in the USA has been described by Novick & Joseph (1991) and Senay et al. (1993), but that intermediate level in the USA actually more closely resembles standard UK clinic treatment, with appointments and urine testing approximately monthly. There is a definite tendency for urine testing to be neglected in unsupervised primary care treatment and, for our part, we recommend that monthly samples should be a minimum requirement for patients on methadone.

In the UK one of the most highly regarded schemes is that in Glasgow (Gruer et al. 1997), in which a secondary service run by general physicians undertakes some treatment and also supervises outright primary care. Transfer is made easy between the secondary service and patients' own practitioners, and all treatment must adhere to set protocols, with incentive payments for physicians only given if this is the case. Counselling and social support are provided, and a notable feature of the scheme is that the majority of patients have supervised consumption of methadone in community pharmacies (Scott 1996). The structured systems of treatment and an associated training programme have proved popular with the general practitioners, 75 of whom were recruited into the scheme over the first two years. This work and other determined approaches to involving general practitioners in drug misuse treatment (Greenwood 1996) have demonstrated that the undoubted problems can be overcome, provided there is a mechanism for overall coordination, a route into secondary treatment for more problematic patients, and suitable emphasis on security of treatment.

## Summary

In countries where drug misuse treatment is very restricted, there are often calls for it to be broadened to more general medical practice. In the UK there are few restrictions, and therefore much experience with treatment in primary care.

The prevalence of drug misuse in the UK is such that the primary care option must be utilized, and there are many examples of good practice. The relative lack of security of the setting, however, leaves it very open to exploitation, and it is common for drug misusers to opportunistically obtain unjustified prescriptions or to take advantage of relatively unstructured treatment. Surveys of primary care physicians show that most are relatively unwilling to offer treatment because of the difficulties encountered, although that situation may be changing with improved training. Those who offer methadone in particular may face unmanageable demand, and restrictions within a practice on numbers taken on for treatment often become necessary.

Treatment in primary care is not just about prescribing methadone, and the setting has advantages for various aspects of early management and associated health care. Liaison work to facilitate general practice treatment has become an important element of drug service provision, this usually being a clinical role which includes providing counselling and monitoring for primary care patients. Particularly where there are waiting lists for clinics, this combination offers the opportunity for early detoxification regimes, including lofexidine for heroin users, as well as longer-term treatment.

Stabilized methadone patients can be transferred to primary care, provided adequate monitoring is in place. Secondary services operated by the physicians may be able to see large numbers of such patients, including those whose own doctor is unwilling to provide treatment. The scheme in Glasgow has been particularly successful in both providing a practitioner-led secondary service and encouraging outright primary care treatment, with aspects such as easy transfer of patients, set protocols and associated training probably enhancing the acceptability of involvement for doctors.

# 7

# Balancing security and accessibility

## Introduction

In community treatment of drug misuse at any level, there is an ever-present need to balance the safety and security of treatments against not only their general effectiveness but also their ability to attract and retain users on a significant scale. The issues relate most acutely to the prescribing of substitution treatments, given the risks inherent in this approach but also the proven ability of methadone in particular to encourage presentation to services. In recent years the harm-reduction and possible HIV-preventive benefits of methadone treatment have been emphasized, and services have placed a premium on accessibility and user-friendliness, with relaxation of the rules and regulations of treatment in many cases. This process, and issues of effectiveness, have been discussed in Chapter 1, but here we should examine the other side of the equation relating to safety, which is receiving increasing attention for various reasons, including medico-legal sensitivity.

The dilemma for those providing treatment services is as follows. Given the nature of drug misuse, and the nature of substitution treatments within drug misuse, a proportion of patients will manipulate the treatment system and abuse the medications, if given the chance. The only way to (virtually) eliminate such abuse, apart from the untenable position of avoiding such treatments altogether, is to require all patients to attend a dispensing centre every day for supervised consumption of methadone. Such a restrictive approach leads to two main criticisms: first, that individuals cannot normalize their lifestyle if faced with such requirements and, secondly, that management of this kind is likely to deter the most severe cases, who may especially need treatment and may pose the highest risks to the community. The ideological swing of the pendulum within half a decade, towards very accessible and relatively undemanding treatment at the height of the concerns about HIV transmission, and then to more secure and restrictive treatment after various problems became evident, is reflected in the recommendations of the UK's main advisory body on drug misuse (Advisory Council on the Misuse of Drugs 1988,

1993, Raistrick 1994). Although, as previously noted, there is much variation internationally in the delivery of methadone treatment, these broad trends have occurred in many countries (Farrell et al. 1995), and they will now be examined.

## The changing policy picture

The present move to more restrictive methadone policies essentially means that services have come full circle, as these were usual before the changes brought about by the HIV agenda. The 1988 report referred to above (Advisory Council on the Misuse of Drugs 1988) concerned policies which would be effective in preventing the spread of HIV, and generally lamented the difficulties in obtaining methadone treatment in the UK, and also the tendency for patients to be routinely discharged from prescribing regimes if they continued to use illicit drugs. It was felt that such limited and universally demanding treatment would not assist a sufficiently wide range of addicts in order to make an impact in public health terms, and recommended fundamental changes in the philosophy of services. Thus, the report stated that 'services must now make contact with as many of the hidden population of drug misusers as possible' and that 'we must be prepared to work with those who continue to misuse drugs to help them reduce the risks involved in doing so', and prescribing was very much involved in those two aims. In particular, a patient on prescribed methadone should be retained if there was movement towards any of a 'range of acceptable goals', which could include stopping sharing injecting equipment, stopping injecting, or a reduction in other drug use rather than simply abstinence from all other drugs in all cases. As part of making treatment more 'flexible', dispensing increasingly occurred at local community pharmacies convenient for each patient, with no particular requirement that this had to be on a daily basis.

These various aspects were not revolutionary in the UK, as many clinicians already recognized that some flexibility in methadone treatment was necessary to enable benefits to occur in patients in very different individual circumstances. However, the principle of methadone *replacing* heroin use is a fairly fundamental one, whether based on the model of narcotic blockade (see Chapter 1), the principle of behavioural shaping, or straightforward safety concerns about combining the two drugs, and so the advice to avoid discharging patients for additional drug use is inherently controversial. Generally speaking, many of the principles of flexible and 'low-threshold' treatment were widely adopted in Europe (e.g. Buning et al. 1990, Klingemann 1996, Plomp et al. 1996), but there has been more adherence to the original model of highly structured and demanding methadone programmes in the USA, based on the strength of the supporting evidence (Ball & Ross 1991). While nearly all the formal advisory recommendations regarding prescribing in this period mainly encouraged the use of oral methadone, the principles of flexible treatment and retaining difficult individuals clearly also underlie the experimental use in some European schemes of injectable drugs or alternative opiates such as diamorphine, for committed injectors (Metrebian et al. 1996, Uchtenhagen et al. 1996).

It is very difficult to establish how successful the pragmatic expansion of flexible methadone prescribing has been and, furthermore, whether the benefits outweigh the disadvantages. The availability of methadone and its role in encouraging users to attend services, where they can obtain clean injecting equipment and receive other harm-reduction advice, are considered to be partly responsible for the rate of HIV infection in drug misusers in the UK being so low (Stimson 1996). Anonymous testing in England, apart from London, indicates an overall HIV prevalence rate of under 1% in injecting drug users, and this outcome, following the initially very high rates in some parts of the UK, has been described as 'a stupendous public health achievement' (Wodak 1996). It now transpires that, in addition to the known high rates of hepatitis B (Farrell et al. 1990), large proportions of many populations of injecting drug users have hepatitis C (Waller & Holmes 1995, Wodak 1997, Serfaty et al. 1997), the higher infectivity of this agent probably having resulted in transmission through various kinds of equipment sharing which were not sufficient to transmit HIV and were not so clearly advised against as actual sharing of needles (Wells 1998).

Of the various elements of the HIV-preventive approach, however, the specific effects of the increased flexibility in methadone prescribing have not themselves been studied (Stimson 1996), and meanwhile various problems relating to the departure from the more rigid systems have become evident. These mainly concern aspects of abuse and diversion of medication and, even though the general harm-reduction picture appears very encouraging, it was probably inevitable that some reaction in terms of methadone policies would come. The 1993 advisory report for the UK (Advisory Council on the Misuse of Drugs 1993) therefore included 'a re-examination of substitute prescribing', noting that 'since the publication of our [previous] report, there has been a substantial expansion in the availability of substitute prescribing, [and] there is now a need to examine closely the framework in which this treatment is delivered'. It was suggested that having a range of acceptable goals of prescribing could lead to unsatisfactory treatment: 'our first report highlighted the usefulness of intermediate goals ... while this provided a framework for considering models of intervention, there has been concern about the position of drug users who become stuck for a prolonged period at an intermediate goal ... as a result, treatment interventions often lack any clear aim or focus, goals are rarely reviewed and mechanisms for monitoring and exit to detoxification programs are poorly articulated [and] we are concerned that such prescribing could be having little impact on drug use or risk-taking behaviour'. There were then a series of recommendations for what can be termed a general 'tightening-up' of methadone treatment, in terms of patient selection, organization, treatment delivery and monitoring.

Various theoretical and practical problems which arise in the course of providing realistic methadone treatment have been discussed in Chapters 1 and 3, and the security issue is as difficult to manage as any. As so often it is necessary to tread something of a middle path, in this case between the most restrictive and the most liberal programmes, and a highly authoritative international review concluded that 'it is likely that policy analysts and treatment providers in countries with high levels of regulation and structured programs will press for reduction in constraints, whereas settings such as Britain with minimal structure will move in the direction of more formalised delivery systems' (Farrell et al. 1994). This is more than a matter of mere ideology, as the reverse side of the coin from greater accessibility is represented by some of the problems which can most bring drug services into disrepute. A very gloomy picture of methadone treatment was portrayed in the study by Payne-James et al. (1994), who interviewed almost 150 consecutive drug misusers who were held in police custody in London. Nearly half had been involved in treatment at some stage, with one-third being on methadone or other prescribed drugs at the time of arrest. The vast majority of those individuals were using drugs in addition to their prescription, and indeed there was no difference in the amount of money spent on drugs between those who were on prescriptions and those who were not. The authors acknowledged that as police surgeons they would see a somewhat unrepresentative sample of users, but concluded that 'it is quite clear that if one of the aims [of methadone] is to replace illicit drugs use, the effectiveness of such programmes appears virtually non-existent in this study population. As has been observed previously it appears that the prescribed drug is commonly sold to finance buying the drugs that are really wanted.' Similar reservations have been expressed in Australia by White (1994), who reviewed various studies showing high levels of ongoing crime and drug misuse by those in methadone treatment, and found in his own audits that methadone only benefitted the small minority of patients who were well motivated.

Guarding against problems of abuse of treatment might be considered justification enough to adopt restrictive policies in methadone programmes. In general, no treatment services should be interested in individuals who sell their medication, or alter prescriptions, and if patients are found to be doing this their places can go immediately to others who are waiting. Looking a little bit deeper, is the argument about severe cases being deterred by restrictive approaches also a spurious one? If an individual is not prepared to accept certain limitations which go with controlled drug treatment, are they likely to be too unreasonable or too unmotivated to benefit? It is not possible to answer that question definitively, but the assumption during the period of expansion of pragmatic treatment, backed up by the experiences of those within the better programmes, has been that there is a group of individuals who cannot comply with treatment conditions which might be considered theoretically the most desirable, but who make genuine clinical progress when there is some relaxation in the approach. It is that view which is increasingly being tested, in the light of the discrepancy between the systematic evidence for structured and unstructured treatment which still remains, the disturbing reports of uncontrolled situations as referred to above, the lessening of the HIV threat which prompted the change to low-threshold treatment, and other factors. The most serious adverse consequence which can occur as a result of unsupervised treatment is that an individual may die from an overdose of their own or somebody else's medication, and it may be decided to restrict all treatment – more than would be necessary for most individuals – simply to prevent this possibility. Deaths from treatment medications have received much publicity, and this aspect will now be considered.

## Drug misuse deaths

Deaths from treatment medications must be put into context, the first point being that any treatment for drug misuse is a response to a condition which itself has a high mortality rate. Rates vary widely between different populations depending on various factors, notably including the local prevalence of HIV, but several studies have shown that between 1 and 3% of drug misusers die each year (Oppenheimer et al. 1994, Goedert et al. 1995, Darke & Zador 1996, Fugelstadt et al. 1997, Frischer et al. 1997). Studies inevitably have mainly been of cohorts who were originally identified from treatment services, but many individuals drop out of treatment and so the findings from the long-term follow-ups can be considered semi-naturalistic. In one such cohort of 4200 injecting drug users in Rome, the cumulative risk of death by the age of 40 was 29.3% (Davoli et al. 1997). These kinds of rates have been variously considered to be between 6 and 22 times those expected in the same age group in the general population (Oppenheimer et al. 1994, Goedert et al. 1995, Darke & Zador 1996, Frischer et al. 1997).

The main causes of death are infections, HIV, accidents, violence, overdoses, and other self-harm (Frischer et al. 1993, Goedert et al. 1995, Fugelstadt et al. 1995, Darke & Zador 1996, Farrell et al. 1996). Within overdoses, it is notoriously difficult to separate suicidal attempts from accidental overdosage (Davoli et al. 1993), but the latter was considered to account for 47% of deaths of injecting drug users in one study in Glasgow (Frischer et al. 1993). The classic risky situation is when a user returns to taking his or her previously typical amount when the tolerance has reduced through being off drugs for a period, but also particularly pure street heroin may be encountered, and other risk factors such as additional alcohol use have been identified (Farrell et al. 1996). Although many of the drugs of misuse are known to cause fatalities, in most areas where opiates are used the overwhelming majority of drug-related deaths are in those who misuse opiates by injection. The only major exceptions to this pattern are in areas where there is a high prevalence of use of crack cocaine, so that a study in New York City found that cocaine, often with secondary use of opiates and alcohol, caused almost three-quarters of fatal drug overdoses (Tardiff et al. 1996).

In keeping with the general rise in illicit drug use, rates of drug-related deaths have been shown to be increasing in many countries (Wysowski et al. 1993, Risser & Schneider 1994, Bentley & Busuttil 1996, Davoli et al. 1997). Much controversy has surrounded the deaths from methadone (Drummer et al. 1992, Clark et al. 1995, Bentley & Busuttil 1996), as inevitably additional issues are raised when a treatment drug appears to be responsible, and there are policy implications for services, of the kind referred to above. Supporters of flexible methadone treatment claim not only that the rising trend in virtually all indicators of drug misuse is bound to also apply to the abuse of methadone if treatment is extended sufficiently but, more constructively, that there should be a dynamic relationship whereby recruitment into methadone treatment can reduce the likelihood of death from heroin. In their brief review of suicide and overdose among opiate addicts, Farrell et al. (1996) state simply that 'methadone maintenance appears to protect against death from overdose', citing a study by Capelhorn et al. (1994). In this long-term follow-up of Australian methadone patients, it was found that subjects were nearly three times as likely to die outside of methadone maintenance as in it, and additional data showed that discharge from treatment had itself been more likely at relatively low methadone doses, and in abstinence-oriented treatment. It appears, therefore, that the opiate users at highest risk may be those who are not only dependent enough to require methadone, but who also have difficulty complying with treatment, perhaps because of inadequate dosing. The authors of the study believe that 'in order to minimise heroin addicts' risk of death they should be offered indefinite, high-dose methadone maintenance', but that policy can itself only be safely adopted if the treatment conditions are secure. It is of interest that in the large study by Fugelstadt et al. (1997), which involved a follow-up period of eight years and included 222 addicts who had received methadone treatment, no deaths occurred among HIV-negative subjects who were participating in the strictly regulated methadone programme.

One major problem regarding methadone treatment is that there is substantial overlap between dosages which are clinically necessary for some individuals, and those which may be fatal in others. In fact, more than that, the blood methadone concentrations which it is claimed are necessary for proper clinical benefit (Dole 1988, Loimer et al. 1991b) are similar to those which many laboratories class as fatal levels (Worm et al. 1993, Clark et al. 1995). In the same way with heroin, Darke et al. (1997) found a substantial overlap between blood morphine concentrations in deaths attributed to heroin overdose and in 100 current heroin users. A third of current users had morphine concentrations over twice the toxic blood morphine concentration employed by the analytical laboratories, and 7% had morphine levels higher than the median recorded for fatal cases. However, alcohol was detected in half of the fatal cases but in only one current heroin user, and there was a significant negative correlation among fatal cases between blood morphine and blood alcohol concentrations. There was no difference between the groups in the proportions testing positive for blood benzodiazepines.

With methadone deaths, there is no strong evidence to suggest that a particular sensitivity to the drug accounts for deaths at relatively low blood concentration levels, and the general pattern of risk would appear to be similar to that in heroin use. Thus, particular risks are posed when an ordinary amount of methadone is taken by an individual who is not tolerant to the drug, or whose tolerance has reduced, or when other drugs or alcohol are additionally taken. Clark et al. (1995) reported 18 deaths from methadone poisoning which occurred between 1991 and 1994 in Sheffield, noting that only three of the people were long-term methadone users. Eight had obtained methadone illegally, while seven cases appeared to illustrate the risk which is present at the time of initiating methadone treatment, in that they died within 1–4 days of starting the drug. Furthermore, other drugs were present in all but two cases, one of whom was a tragic case of a three-year-old girl who had been forced to take methadone. The additional drugs – benzodiazepines, morphine, cyclizine and amphetamine – were present in low concentrations, and the authors, who are forensic pathologists, were confident that in these deaths methadone was the main cause. Not surprisingly, they recommended that there should be caution when prescribing methadone to new patients, and consideration given to controlled administration. Worm et al. (1993) reported an increase in methadone deaths with a very similar pattern in Copenhagen, with only half the individuals having been in methadone treatment, and morphine, benzodiazepines and alcohol also commonly found. Capelhorn (1998) studied deaths which occurred in the initial stages of methadone treatment in New South Wales, Australia, calculating a rate of fatal iatrogenic methadone toxicity of 2.2 per thousand admissions to methadone maintenance.

In general, it seems that once tolerance to methadone is established, very high doses can safely be taken by individuals in treatment, provided they do not increase their risk by taking additional drugs. In their brief report which criticizes the criteria adopted by pathologists in attributing deaths to methadone, Merrill et al. (1996) describe an error by a community pharmacist which resulted in three methadone patients receiving ten times their normal daily dose, all of whom survived. Certainly it is common to be told in a clinic – often in the context of complaints about the noneuphoriant effect of methadone – that 'I could take 300 ml and still not feel anything', and there has been experimentation of ultra-high dose treatment in some secure settings.

The steps which can be taken by a treatment service to reduce the risk of methadone deaths in particular have been indicated, including cautious initial prescribing, daily dispensing, supervised consumption, controls and limits in prescribing of any additional drugs, and screening for other drug or alcohol misuse. More generally, because opiate overdoses are often witnessed by other drug users, there have been calls for users to be instructed in preventive aspects. On interviewing 329 heroin users regarding nonfatal heroin overdoses, Darke et al. (1996a) found that 68% had previously overdosed, with the majority of the most recent overdoses also involving other central nervous system depressants (alcohol, benzodiazepines and other opioids). Overdoses were associated with longer heroin careers, greater dependence and higher levels of alcohol consumption, while Risser & Schneider (1994) found that alcohol use was itself strongly associated with higher age in a study of fatalities. Darke et al. (1996b) also report that 86% of their 329 users had witnessed heroin overdose, on an average of six occasions, and it is this situation which raises the possibility of instructing users in resuscitation techniques, or even in the use of naloxone (Strang & Farrell 1992). There have not so far been wide initiatives in this area, and many difficulties are obvious, including the fine distinction between desired heroin intoxication and an 'overdose', and possible impairment of associated users. Darke et al. (1996b) found that users who had witnessed overdoses had typically been reluctant to call for an ambulance, apparently because of fear of police involvement, but were keen in principle on the idea of having naloxone available.

The issue of drug-related deaths is only one of many which needs to be considered in judging appropriate treatment responses in drug misuse, but it is bound to weigh particularly heavily because of its nature. We will consider the main implications which the situations relating to deaths have for services, taking into account the wider picture as far as possible.

## Implications for services

Although the occurrence of deaths involving methadone can place those providing services in an awkward position, a strong defence can be made for the use of this drug in treatment. In addition to the study by Capelhorn et al. (1994) referred to above, several other studies have shown methadone treatment to have a beneficial effect in reducing drug misuse deaths. Gearing (1977) reported a 0.8% mortality rate among 3000 subjects in methadone programmes compared with an 8.3% death rate in heroin addicts who were offered detoxification only, and in Sweden, Gronbladh et al. (1990) demonstrated that death rates not only reduced in methadone maintenance but returned to high levels in patients expelled from the programme. Fugelstadt et al. (1995) found a three times relative risk of overdose death for opiate misusers who had never been in methadone maintenance, relative to those currently in maintenance treatment, while Zador et al. (1996) found that only 2% of heroin-related deaths in 1992 in New South Wales, Australia, were in methadone maintenance at the time of death, and 75% had never been in methadone treatment. There are many possible relationships and confounding factors here, including a tendency for the worst-risk individuals to either not seek treatment or not be able to comply, but an important factor in terms of treatment programmes is that these results all related to generally strict methadone regimes. Indeed, from the literature it appears that providing methadone in the model of the original highly-structured programmes (see Chapter 2) would go a long way to reducing methadone deaths and overall drug deaths, with high dosage proving beneficial in reducing discharge rates (Capelhorn et al. 1994) and the consequent risks.

It is extremely unlikely, however, that there will be a widespread return to highly structured methadone programmes, even with the general move towards making treatment more secure. In many countries there has been more than a decade of considering methadone as realistically a partial treatment, which reduces other drug use and promotes engagement with services, and the principles of continuing to prescribe for some who still use heroin, and responding to polydrug users, have become firmly established. For logistical and security reasons such approaches actually require lower methadone dosages, and we have discussed the somewhat circular arguments whereby dosing in such treatment can be considered inadequate, but if discharge does occur from higher-dose but stricter programmes, the outcomes may be worst of all. In terms of risk of methadone deaths, and diversion of medication and general abuse of treatment, the worst combination is to accept the arguments for both high-dose methadone *and* the principles of flexible treatment, for instance accommodating infrequent dispensing or some additional drug use. This would seem to be asking for trouble, but the arguments for both are often made strongly, and not necessarily independently.

If some flexibility in treatment is to be retained, in dispensing arrangements and other related aspects, there is a great advantage in using a substitute medication which cannot itself be fatal. Because of combined opiate agonist and antagonist properties, buprenorphine appears to fulfil this criterion (Mello & Mendelson 1985), and the possible benefits of this drug over methadone have been discussed in Chapter 2. There is still risk from use in combination with sedative drugs (Reynaud et al. 1998), although in the case of some euphoriant drugs such as cocaine the properties of buprenorphine may actually make combined usage less likely (Foltin & Fischman 1996). As buprenorphine is introduced more into clinical practice, the relative safety of the drug is likely to become an important issue; in the UK some areas have had a substantial history of injected abuse of buprenorphine, and it has even been suggested that the prescribing controls which were brought in as a response may actually have contributed to a rise in drug misuse deaths in one such area, as addicts turned to more dangerous alternatives (Hammersley et al. 1995).

The security issues relating to the other newer alternative substitution agent, levo-alpha-acetylmethadol (LAAM), are similar to those with methadone, which it resembles in all properties other than its longer duration of action. This longer action could pose a particular risk in those prone to using additional drugs, and LAAM should be seen as mainly indicated for well-motivated patients (Ling et al. 1994). One of the keenest proponents of diamorphine prescribing, Marks (1994), published an analysis of figures from UK Home Office literature, apparently showing methadone to cause proportionately many more fatalities than 'street' heroin, but the calculation can be criticized for depending on notoriously unreliable drugs notification patterns, and so far there is no comparable information on the safety of diamorphine as a treatment drug, or the other opiates which are sometimes advocated.

Although changes in the culture of treatment take time, the shift in emphasis towards treating better-motivated and more compliant individuals is clearly apparent in the UK currently. We have noted elsewhere that part of the change within services is due to the demands of large numbers of young heroin users, who neither want nor require substitution treatment, but in relation to methadone, the policy changes are being put into place as recommended in the later report of the Advisory Council on the Misuse of Drugs (1993) and subsequent national treatment guidelines. The period of most open access to treatment and most toleration of the range of motivation was marked by the threat of HIV; now injecting drug misusers are found to have high rates of hepatitis C, but the risk of spread to the general heterosexual population is not as great, and so it is suspected that the policy arguments will not be as forceful (Wells 1998). Of the main rationales for not insisting on restrictive – and therefore secure – treatment conditions in all cases, the social argument of enabling normalization of lifestyle has perhaps worn rather thin, with clinicians observing that this does not necessarily occur even with the easier conditions, and that time freed-up by not attending for dispensing is often not spend constructively. The argument that restrictive treatment deters severe cases carries more force, especially where – as commonly occurs – difficult individuals simply exploit primary care treatment if the local specialist service tightens up its conditions.

There will always be drug misusers whose treatment needs are not easily met, and their management should mainly be within specialist services. It must be recognized, however, that the retention in such services of individuals with severe personality disorder or mental illness, or who continue to use illicit drugs, raises various additional problematic issues, including those of a medico-legal nature. Even though retention may often seem preferable to the alternative, the most extreme individuals present the highest risks not only for fatalities, but for other kinds of behavioural disturbance and drug-related incidents, within or outside clinics, which may have implications for service providers. There may therefore be a group who are considered 'too hot to handle' in view of the prevailing medico-legal climate and trends such as comparative monitoring of adverse incidents between services. It seems clear that unless appropriate adjustments and allowances are made, some discharges could be due to defensive practice in these areas. The distinction between axis-I mental illness – particularly psychosis – and personality disorder can be important to draw in determining individual responsibility for problematic behaviours in such circumstances. In any situations where direct treatment is withdrawn, basic harm-reduction facilities, including clean injecting equipment, must remain available.

The dilemma regarding severe cases is illustrated by a trend in the drug misuse deaths in Sheffield. The series referred to above (Clark et al. 1995), which immediately pre-dated my own involvement in treatment, included several young people who had died as a result of experimenting with diverted methadone. It was made a priority to eliminate such deaths, and so the security of treatment was generally enhanced, with the effect – among others – that it became much more difficult to buy methadone on the streets. Recently, this type of death has not occurred, but there have been a small number of other deaths of patients in treatment, all individuals with broadly similar histories. They have been around 30 years of age, polydrug users of long standing, and acknowledged to be extremely difficult to manage, with ongoing additional drug use on top of methadone treatment. Again, treatment had been made as secure as possible under UK conditions, while the argument to retain them in treatment just won over the case for discharging them for noncompliance, which would definitely have occurred in the original model of methadone pro-grammes. In turn they died of multiple drug ingestion, and even though it is possible – perhaps likely – that we actually prolonged their lives, nevertheless they represent deaths in our service, with all the implications that that has in service scrutiny. In blunt terms such patients represent something of a liability, and services generally may become less willing to have such difficult cases in treatment, on clinical and medico-legal grounds. It is of interest that in the study by Worm et al. (1993) from Copenhagen, the average age of individuals dying from methadone overdosage increased over time, perhaps partly indicating a similar group to the fatalities we have seen.

The increased sensitivity about methadone deaths is demonstrated in the conclusion by Capelhorn (1998), who found a low rate of iatrogenic methadone toxicity but recommended that patients should be informed of the risks and give written consent to methadone treatment, and that there should be a medical assessment each day during the first 1–2 weeks of treatment.

## Summary

In providing services for drug misusers, issues to do with delivery of treatment are generally as important to consider as selection of treat-ments themselves. A highly problematic area is the delivery of substitu-tion treatments, since the nature of this approach means that they will be abused by a proportion of individuals presenting. The original type of methadone programmes devised in the USA allowed for very little abuse of medication, as there was supervised consumption of methadone for each patient every day on clinic premises. In addition, methadone could not contribute to potentially dangerous multiple drug-taking, as those with a tendency to polydrug use were usually not considered suitable in the first place, and if additional drug use occurred once on methadone, a patient would be discharged from treatment.

As discussed in Chapter 1, methadone treatment has moved a long way from that model, and the emphasis on accessibility of treatment, and retention of individuals in the face of some ongoing drug misuse, has undoubtedly compromised the security aspects. These policies emerged as methadone treatment was expanded when drug misusers became implicated in the HIV epidemic, the view being that some relaxation of the original approach was necessary to enable large numbers of users to benefit and reduce risk behaviours, even if only partially. The extent to which this pragmatic approach to methadone prescribing has helped contain the HIV epidemic is open to debate, but this period has highlighted the difficulties in striking an appropriate balance in treatment between security and safety on the one hand, and accessibility and flexibility on the other. Inevitably there is now something of a backlash in policy terms, with the problems resulting from diversion of medication in flexible services having become particularly apparent.

An issue which assumes an importance which is out of proportion to its rate of occurrence is that of drug misuse deaths. These have generally risen along with many other indicators of drug misuse in countries across the world, but there is particular sensitivity if the deaths involve the treatment drugs, primarily methadone. Some types of methadone death clearly reflect the changes in treatment policies, including nontolerant individuals who misrepresent their drug use and too readily obtain methadone from an accessible service, patients who continue to use drugs alongside methadone and die of multiple overdose, and those who obtain diverted methadone. Strong supporters of methadone treatment point to evidence that deaths are actually more likely in opiate misusers who are not engaged in such treatment, but the studies which have shown this relate to methadone programmes with relatively strict treatment conditions. The 'protective' effect of methadone against drug misuse deaths is clearly not a straightforward one, as although it enables reduction or elimination of other drug misuse in many individuals across various types of programme, it can also constitute the direct means to fatally overdose. The alternative substitution agent, buprenorphine, is of considerable interest in that regard, as it appears impossible to fatally overdose by taking that drug alone.

Although it is likely that the overall benefits of flexible methadone treatment have been substantial, many prescribing services are presently moving towards a more restrictive approach. From a perspective of the history of methadone treatment, this can be seen as an inevitable swing of the pendulum, in which the problems of successive models of providing methadone have become apparent in turn, but there is increasingly the additional consideration of medico-legal sensitivity. There are high degrees of risk involved in drug misuse treatment, which must be acknowledged and addressed not only by clinicians in direct case management, but by treatment service employers and legal advisors.

# 8

## Dual diagnosis – drug misuse and psychiatric disorder

### Introduction

One of the reasons why drug misuse is managed substantially as a psychiatric specialty is that it is strongly associated with various pervasive and clinically important psychiatric conditions. Studies have examined the relationship both ways round – that is, investigating rates of mental disorders in drug misusers, or the extent of drug misuse in mentally ill populations, and some of these are discussed here. In practice, clinicians must be skilled in recognizing personality disorder (often as a continuation of adolescent conduct disorder), depression, and anxiety states, all of which are extremely common and need to be distinguished from the effects of drug misuse itself. Personality disorder is particularly important, as it is often the main cause of abnormal mood in drug misusers and it exerts strong negative effects on many forms of treatment; the first part of the chapter focuses on this and the difficult area of drug-induced psychosis. The rest of the chapter is then given over to a discussion from the other perspective, of substance misuse problems in those with severe mental illness, as the rising rates of such problems are currently posing great difficulties in the provision of general psychiatric treatment in the community.

The management of those with schizophrenia and other psychotic conditions who misuse drugs is highly problematic, partly because such individuals do not comply well with conventional addiction treatment approaches, and a literature is emerging on ultra-specialist services for that group. A wider difficulty is that the drugs involved tend not to be opiates, and so even if engagement is encouraged, there are few specific drug misuse treatments which can be applied. If only because of the particular vulnerability of those with severe mental illness, however, and the propensity of various drugs to worsen psychosis, such users need to be accorded some priority in services, especially those which are psychiatrically based. The case for ultra-specialist services for this group is arguable, but some fundamental treatment principles which have been identified from such services are examined here, and appear to have general applicability. In most areas there is no special service provision, and much reliance needs to be placed on good liaison between general psychiatric and drug misuse teams.

In terms of overall prevalence, the Epidemiologic Catchment Area (ECA) study of over 20 000 subjects in the community found a 53% lifetime prevalence of nonsubstance-related mental disorder in those with drug dependence or abuse (Regier et al. 1990). This is actually a lower figure than in most clinical studies, probably because of the broader population and also the limited inclusion of personality disorders in the community study method. The other way round, a 15% lifetime history of drug dependence or abuse was found in those with nonsubstance-related mental disorders, rising to 28% in those with schizophrenia.

## Mental disorders in drug misusers

In the ECA study the most common psychiatric conditions in those with drug dependence or abuse were anxiety disorders (28%), affective disorders (26%), antisocial personality disorder (ASPD) (18%) and schizophrenia (7%). Studies in clinical settings (Rounsaville et al. 1982, Ross et al. 1988, Darke et al. 1994c) also indicate high rates of depression, various anxiety disorders and ASPD, plus other substance misuse and psychosexual dysfunction. It can clearly be seen that all these conditions have features which require separation from the effects of drugs (e.g. anxiety, psychosis, sexual problems), withdrawal effects (anxiety from sedatives, depression from stimulants), and other aspects of drug taking. Standard treatment approaches are indicated for diagnosed disorders broadly as in nondrug misusers but, in practice, drug misusers tend to comply poorly with nonpharmacological treatments. For depression, there is a particular case for using the specific serotonergic re-uptake inhibitors such as fluoxetine or sertraline, as they may have additional effects in reducing drug craving (Sellers et al. 1991), and in improving some aspects of personality disorder (see below), as well as being well tolerated. For anxiety disorders it will usually be desired to avoid benzodiazepines, but this is discussed further in the section on benzodiazepines in Chapter 2. When it is felt that psychological counselling is indicated, given its general benefits in neurotic conditions, the most practical option is often to include aspects such as anxiety management within drug counselling sessions from a drug team's community psychiatric nurses.

There are some general influences on clinical features and progress which are quite characteristic of drug misusers. Often there are high rates of adverse life events, reflecting the direct and indirect complications of a drug-using lifestyle, as well as an effect of personality disorder (Seivewright 1987, Poulton & Andrews 1992). It must not be assumed that consequences such as adjustment reactions will follow, as drug misusers can appear to take many types of events in their stride, but sometimes the psychiatric effects are significant and this possibility must be anticipated. Impulsive reactions to events are an important factor in self-harm in this population, who have ready access to dangerous methods (Farrell et al. 1996). Personality disorder and depression are both related to self-harm, while general effects of personality disorder are to increase levels of neurotic symptoms (Tyrer et al. 1990) and impair response to psychiatric treatments (Reich & Vasile 1993). Importantly, studies have shown improvements in psychological disorders such as anxiety and depressive states on methadone maintenance treatment (Musselman & Kell 1995). This raises the question (as discussed in Chapter 1) of the mechanism by which methadone produces its benefits, but broadly it would seem that in some cases psychological symptoms are due to drug use and the various associated lifestyle problems. The clinical message is that if moderate depressive or other neurotic features are encountered in the context of starting methadone treatment, the effects of stabilization should usually be awaited before considering specific psychiatric treatments. Also, there can be great improvements in psychological state following detoxification from drugs (Craig et al. 1990).

Clinicians are sometimes required to make a judgement as to whether drug misuse or a psychiatric disorder is the 'primary' condition, especially where that determines which type of service initially manages an individual. An example might be an amphetamine user whose drug taking seems linked with problems of depression and lack of confidence. Approaches take into account which condition came first, and careful teasing out of symptoms, but it is also necessary to decide which is currently the major contributor to an individual's various difficulties. In that respect there is a wide spectrum, and certainly those whose drug use is low level or well controlled can feel aggrieved when 'all my problems get put down to drugs'. Nevertheless, established drug use tends to exert a powerful influence on an individual's situation and needs, and drug services should, in practical terms, usually operate a low threshold for becoming involved with cases in which it is present to any significant degree. In opiate misusers, nondrug-related counselling or treatment will be unsuccessful if a matter such as consideration for methadone remains unaddressed.

## Personality disorder

In a review of ten years of studies, Verheul et al. (1995) concluded that the best estimate of prevalence of personality disorder in drug misusers was 79%. Most studies were of opiate misusers in treatment, and there is some evidence that the rate is lower across the range of drugs, and outside treatment settings (Seivewright & Daly 1997). The 18% figure found in the ECA study, however, is artificially low, as only a limited range of personality features were rated with the Diagnostic Interview Schedule, which appears to have low validity in drug misusers (Griffin et al. 1987).

Making the diagnosis of personality disorder in drug misusers is problematic, due to the particular difficulties of separating true underlying personality disorder from behaviours which develop as part of drug misuse. Most difficulties are with the antisocial behaviours, such as aggressiveness, irresponsibility or tendency to crime, and even in formal diagnostic systems the situation can become rather tautologous. The required approach in both formal and informal rating is to recognize the particular groupings of features which occur in the main categories (those of ASPD or borderline personality disorder are often very apparent in clinical practice), and to take as much account as possible of behaviours which occur independently of drug misuse or cannot be fully explained by it. This includes behaviours prior to dependent drug use, with for instance a history of rebellious behaviour, school absences and petty crime strongly suggesting conduct disorder as a precursor of adult ASPD. The term 'secondary' ASPD is sometimes used to describe adult antisocial behaviours which are consequent on drug misuse, but even studies which adopt methods to exclude those features find ASPD to be the most frequent underlying personality disorder. With a colleague I recently reviewed this subject, examining not only prevalence and the aspect of rating difficulties, but also the effects of personality disorder on outcome and treatment of drug misuse (Seivewright & Daly 1997). Rates of many medical, psychiatric and social complications appear higher in individuals with personality disorder, even including increased rates of HIV infection (Brooner et al. 1993). In most studies causal direction cannot be definitely inferred, but findings such as more injecting, risk behaviours, depression, social impairment and legal problems have high face validity, and the direction of findings is very consistent.

In reviewing the limited evidence regarding treatment, it appeared that personality disorder had a detrimental effect on the results of treatments aimed at abstinence, but not so marked an effect in methadone maintenance (Gill et al. 1992, Darke et al. 1994b). This is probably because methadone maintenance is, by its nature, a relatively undemanding form of treatment, whereas detoxification, at least in a long-term user, requires more of the personal resources which may be impaired in personality disorder. Certainly, time and again in clinical practice methadone proves to be the most realistic option in opiate users with a significant degree of personality disorder, and antisocial behaviours usually then reduce to some extent. Sometimes it may be felt that the personality disorder should be addressed more directly, in therapy or in residential rehabilitation, but this is less often successful. In terms of other medications, there is some evidence that ASPD features such as impulsivity and aggressiveness may be reduced by fluoxetine (Norden 1989, Markowitz et al. 1991) and sertraline (Kavoussi et al. 1994). This suggests another peripheral indication for serotonergic re-uptake inhibitors in substance misusers, along with the possible effect in reducing drug craving (Sellers et al. 1991), and these drugs would seem a good choice in this population if there are grounds for prescribing anyway for depression.

### Drug-induced psychosis

Another area which poses major problems in diagnosis and management is that of drug-induced psychosis, and a recent editorial in the *British Journal of Psychiatry* has been highly critical of the understanding of this concept (Poole & Brabbins 1996). The authors point out that, although '? drug-induced psychosis' is routinely included in the differential diagnosis in young psychotic patients, the evidence for lasting psychosis caused by drugs is weak. The monograph on amphetamine psychosis by Connell (1958) is frequently cited, but he apparently confirmed to these authors that he is widely misquoted, and that what he demonstrated was that psychotic symptoms precipitated by amphetamines occurred only in relation to intoxication. If the drug is withdrawn, resolution of symptoms can be expected, and one of the criticisms is that enduring functional psychoses are not properly diagnosed in drug misusers, as their condition tends to be automatically attributed to drugs. Certainly it is easy to see how, given the high prevalence of drug use in the community, some usage will be genuinely incidental in cases of other psychotic conditions. Table 8.1 indicates the provisional classification of drug-related psychotic reactions suggested in the editorial 'to introduce clarity into a dangerously confused area', all of which fall short of a true enduring disorder.

The listing of drugs possibly causing each condition is based on the availability of some reasonably direct evidence, while the main clinical message is probably that all the drugs listed, with the exception of the

Table 8.1. *Drug-related psychotic reactions*

| Condition | Possible causative drugs |
|---|---|
| Intoxication mimicking functional psychosis | Stimulants, cannabis, solvents, ecstasy, LSD |
| Pathoplastic reactions in functional psychosis | Stimulants, cannabis |
| Chronic hallucinosis ('flashbacks') | LSD, cannabis |
| Drug-induced relapse of functional psychosis | Stimulants, cannabis |
| Withdrawal states | Barbiturates, benzodiazepines |

Based on Poole & Brabbins (1996)

sedative–hypnotics mentioned in relation to withdrawal, can cause short-lived psychotic reactions, and also worsen an existing psychotic condition. Importantly, this does not include opiates, while cyclizine should probably be added (see Chapter 4). Paranoid ideation following amphetamine or cocaine use is well known, and is typically recognized by users as indicating that they should terminate that episode of usage. The reactions with solvents and LSD are more organic in nature, with visual illusions and hallucinations, and the phenomenon of 'flashbacks' is reasonably well documented with LSD in particular. With the sedative–hypnotics, psychotic symptoms appear in the withdrawal state rather than as an intoxication effect, although high-dose misuse can cause confusion and disturbed behaviour. In addition to these conditions, prolonged psychotic reactions may occur when use of the implicated drug itself is ongoing, and such situations can be very troublesome and intractable in clinical practice.

Management has usually been considered to comprise two elements, namely cessation of the drug of misuse and standard antipsychotic drug treatment, as dictated by symptoms. The first can be difficult to achieve, and admission to a psychiatric unit may be necessary to attempt to ensure this (there is still no guarantee), or because of severity of psychosis. Sometimes it is necessary to treat with antipsychotic medication in the face of some known ongoing drug use, in the hope that the medication effect will be over-riding and that, as insight improves, compliance with advice and treatment will generally be better. Medications which act effectively on paranoid symptoms, or which produce sedation, are often particularly indicated. It appears from case reports in the literature that psychotic reactions to ecstasy may sometimes be particularly resistant to treatment (Solowij 1993). There is speculation that this may be related to the neurotoxic effects of the drug, but there is no direct evidence and, in practice, the same treatment approaches have to be used.

Although criticism of the concept of drug-induced psychosis is clearly justified, it remains possible that a psychosis could be substantially caused by drugs and persist in the absence of drug use. Claims have been made in this regard for cannabis (Andreasson et al. 1987) and, clinically, symptoms sometimes appear to persist for weeks, or even months, after all evidence suggests drug use has stopped. There is no definite consensus as to how long such a period needs to be before symptoms should be considered to indicate a functional psychosis, an area which has been considered by Flaum & Schulz (1996). It may also be that drugs can lead to fuller expression of psychotic features in a case of latent or developing psychosis, or in an individual who is constitutionally susceptible by virtue of family history, but such relationships are difficult to demonstrate, and there is little systematic evidence. Boutros & Bowers (1996) have reviewed the relevant literature and conclude that such a threshold-lowering effect does occur.

## Drug misuse in the severely mentally ill

Particular reasons to account for drug misuse by people with schizophrenia, manic depressive psychosis, and other severe mental illnesses may be classed as broadly social, or individual. As institutionalization decreases there is greater exposure to available drugs in the community; some community placements in cities, and other accommodation which the severely mentally ill may be offered, are in areas of high drug prevalence. Also, people with an obvious vulnerability can be exploited by drug dealers, who may for instance give drugs free initially in order to gain a regular customer over whom they have easy control. At an individual level, a person with severe mental illness is likely to have impairments in the processes of judgement and insight which usually afford some control against drug taking. They may then find that drugs actually alleviate some of their symptoms, with cannabis or heroin perhaps providing some relief from hallucinations or troublesome side-effects of medication, or stimulants giving energy in a person with negative symptoms. Clinicians would normally see this as outweighed by the propensity of drugs to directly worsen psychosis, and the adverse effects on psychiatric treatments, but it can be very difficult to discourage drug use when a patient perceives short-term benefits. It may be possible for some individuals to reproduce symptoms which are pleasurable, or they may value the degree of control over their symptoms which drug use brings. Being part of the drugs scene can provide a social role and opportunities for interaction with people which are otherwise lacking, and it is necessary to counter this by involvement in nondrug-related activities as part of treatment.

As well as these general effects, features which distinguish those among the severely mentally ill who are likely to misuse drugs have been investigated. Mueser et al. (1997) found antisocial personality disorder to be a risk factor, just as it is for developing drug misuse generally (see above). Males are more prone, again reflecting the general pattern in drug misuse, and where females do have dual diagnosis they have been found to have more social contact and fewer legal problems, but more violent victimization and medical illness than men (Brunette & Drake 1997).

We have noted that in the large Epidemiological Catchment Area study in the community (Regier et al. 1990) 28% of those with schizophrenia were found to have drug dependence or abuse, but Galanter et al. (1994) point out that such studies do not reflect the major burden that dual diagnosis patients place upon clinical services. From their perspective in New York they suggest that 'the considerable impact of these patients is better reflected in the prevalence of substance abuse in emergency rooms, psychiatric units, medical services and perinatal programs', with 34% of all general hospital psychiatric admissions in New York State assessed as being dually diagnosed (Haugland et al. 1991). In London, Menezes et al. (1996) assessed all patients with psychotic illness who had had contact with the mental health services in a geographical sector, and found a one-year prevalence rate for any substance problem of 36%. Young male subjects had the highest rates, at 50% in the 20–29 age group for drug misuse alone.

As would be expected, the additional aspect of drug misuse has been shown to complicate the progress of those with severe mental illness, in and outside treatment. Thus, the dually diagnosed have been found to have increased levels of violence (Swanson et al. 1990, Cuffell et al. 1994, Scott et al. 1998), hostile behaviour (Bartels et al. 1991), offending (Lehman et al. 1993a, Scott et al. 1998), family problems (Lehman et al. 1993a), homelessness, various poor prognosis features (Drake & Wallach 1989, Swofford et al. 1996), and movement disorders (Bailey et al. 1997), in comparison with individuals with psychosis only. There is generally poorer compliance with treatments, including antipsychotic medication, but increased use of inpatient services and overall treatment costs (Bartels et al. 1993, Haywood et al. 1995, Menezes et al. 1996). While many of these associated problems may partly reflect lifestyle aspects of drug misuse, or in some cases underlying personality features, direct links between use of drugs and worsening of psychotic conditions are increasingly being demonstrated (Shaner et al. 1995, Boutros & Bowers 1996).

**Principles of treatment**

A group of clinical researchers in New Hampshire, USA, who are highly experienced in the treatment of substance abuse in the severely mentally ill have identified certain key principles of management (Drake et al. 1993), which are shown in Table 8.2. They consider that a special approach is necessary because the severely mentally ill do not identify problems in the same way, they typically have difficulty with addiction treatment approaches, such as group therapy, and there is an ever-present danger that this group fall between two sets of services. Their work is in a unit specifically for dual diagnosis patients, but the principles ring true as being generally applicable in working with this patient group in any setting.

Many will recognize the appropriateness of these suggested measures, especially being flexible in terms of opportunities for contact, helping with practical aspects and activities as far as possible, and ensuring integrated treatment. It is also beneficial to form good links with family, partner or anyone else who provides important support to the patient, as they may help in areas such as detecting drug use, managing medication, or compliance with appointments. As with the patient, a broad approach which addresses practical difficulties as well as the clinical conditions is often valued.

Some of the problems of acceptability and compliance in drug misuse treatment may be less in those countries outside the USA where treatment is more pragmatic, and less uniformly based on the 12-step approach and group therapy, which the severely mentally ill can find off-putting. However, any counselling can be difficult in those with impaired cognitive abilities, and it is unfortunate that there are so few useful pharmacological treatments for nonopiate misuse, which is frequently encountered in this population. If the drug misuse is of opiates, it is tempting to use methadone if only because this facilitates engagement so well, but probably the criteria for maintenance on methadone should be similar to those for anybody else.

Table 8.2. *Principles of treatment of drug misuse in the severely mentally ill*

*Assertive outreach*
Visit at home or other places as necessary. Stress benefits of contact and treatment to patient and significant others

*Close monitoring*
Particularly necessary in difficult cases. Opportunities to do this may be presented by sheltered housing, day hospitals, probation, etc

*Integration*
Liaison between general psychiatric and substance misuse services

*Comprehensiveness*
Address practical issues, e.g. activities, benefits, social skills, as well as clinical disorders

*Stable living situation*
Direct efforts towards this, otherwise progress is unlikely

*Flexibility*
Modify the traditional approach to addiction counselling

*Stage-wise treatment*
Recognize which stage of treatment is applicable – engagement/persuasion/ active treatment/relapse prevention

*Longitudinal perspective*
Recognize that drug misuse is a chronic relapsing disorder

*Optimism*
Counter demoralization among patients, families, and treatment providers

Based on Drake et al. (1993)


## Ultra-specialist treatment services

The same New Hampshire group have described 'continuous treatment teams' (Drake et al. 1996), who solely treat dual diagnosis patients, with 24-hour responsibility for case management. There is a flexible approach to individual and group therapy, the latter being either educational or treatment-oriented in the case of those committed to abstinence. There is a practical focus on social situation, social skills and practical aspects of daily living.

Behaviour therapy techniques have also been used with these dual diagnosis patients, to address symptom management, medication management, recreation and leisure, and social skills (Jerrell & Ridgeley 1995). In New York City there has been a combined service comprising a locked ward, a halfway house, and a day programme, the operation and results of which have been described by Galanter et al. (1994). This work is with a particularly challenging population, mostly disadvantaged minorities, homeless, and using crack cocaine. In the inpatient unit there is a token economy system to encourage compliance and participation in therapy, while other elements of the service include a peer leadership approach, educational groups, 12-step addiction groups, and conventional antipsychotic treatment.

Assessing the effectiveness of ultra-specialist services for dual diagnosis is at an early stage, but the preliminary results of the continuous treatment team approach are encouraging (Drake et al. 1996). Jerrell & Ridgeley (1995) compared three approaches – case management, behaviour therapy, and the 12-step model – at a follow-up of two years, and there was a suggestion, within generally encouraging results over 18 months, that behaviour therapy had the most effect, and 12-step treatment the least. Largely unsuccessful attempts at treatment for this group have included an intensive community-based programme which is viewed as not having included an adequate period of preparation (Lehman et al. 1993b), and a residential programme for frequently relapsing patients (Bartels & Drake 1996).

Johnson (1997) has critically examined whether ultra-specialist services should be adopted outside the USA, in particular in Europe. She points out that such a specialized service covering a large geographical area could cut across some of the strong links formed between psychiatric services and primary care in smaller localities, which is increasingly the approach in community psychiatry in the UK. There is also the common dilemma that the more specialized the unit, the more it may discourage others from attempting treatment at all for that patient group. She concludes that it may be preferable to investigate ways of delivering care for dual diagnosis patients within established community mental health teams rather than to form distinct specialist teams.

**Other treatment**
In areas where an ultra-specialist service is not available, there would seem to be two important aspects to addressing the needs of the severely mentally ill who misuse drugs. One is for general psychiatric and drug misuse services to each be committed to managing such individuals, even

in the presence of the accompanying disorder. The other is to have some members of the drug misuse team take particular responsibility for those with severe mental illness, whether it be the existing psychiatrically qualified members or dedicated dual diagnosis workers.

Although Johnson (1997) says in her review that 'there are few reports of simultaneous delivery of care for both disorders', it is common for individuals to be patients of both psychiatric and drug misuse services. Each service should manage its own element, with mechanisms in place for good liaison. Although there are areas where roles can become blurred, such as attempting to reduce drug misuse in a psychotic condition, or assessing the effects of a period on an antidepressant, in our own services there are no major problems with the provision of ongoing concurrent management. In Sheffield, if a schizophrenic has a problem of drug misuse, the general psychiatric team will undertake management of his or her schizophrenia along standard clinical lines, while our drug service will provide specific drug misuse treatments and all drug-related counselling. If the psychiatric condition becomes acute and requires inpatient treatment, it is recognized that the general psychiatric unit is more appropriate than a drug admission facility, as elements such as high-dose antipsychotic medication, containment of disturbed behaviour or compulsory detention may be required. Conversely, if there needs to be a greater focus on a drug misuse aspect, such as a controlled detoxification, we would undertake that and call upon the general psychiatrists as necessary. There seems to be great variation between other localities as to whether such a system operates well, no doubt reflecting a wide range of factors including the extent of pressure on the facilities involved. Hall & Farrell (1997) point to training in detection of general psychiatric conditions and drug misuse, within the converse services, as a way of improving treatment of comorbid disorders and joint working.

Workers with a remit for dual diagnosis can be attached to either the general psychiatric service or the drug misuse service. The type of caseload they receive will reflect this – more cases of schizophrenia if attached to psychiatry, more personality disorder and depression through the drug service. In Sheffield the priority was first identified within general psychiatry, and two dual diagnosis workers are attached to a community team which specifically provides assertive outreach for those with severe enduring mental health problems. Clinical supervision, however, is from the substance misuse service and the model of working, with small personal caseloads plus a wider role in training to facilitate treatment in other services, derives from the principles of Drake et al. (1993).

## Summary

Drug misuse is by no means exclusively a psychiatric specialty, but the links between it and various psychiatric conditions are very clear. With much current extension of drug misuse treatment to other settings, notably general practice, dual diagnosis patients are likely to be seen as one group suitable for more specialized management, along perhaps with nonresponders and other severe cases or special groups. If personality disorder is included, however, up to 80% of drug misusers have an additional psychiatric diagnosis, and so for practical implementation that principle will have to be watered down to some extent.

Personality disorder is very important to recognize in drug misusers, as the presence of significant antisocial characteristics in particular is consistently associated with high rates of complications and poor response to drug misuse treatment. The latter effect applies especially to treatments aimed at full detoxification, with personality disorder possibly less of a problem in the relatively undemanding approach of methadone maintenance. Many behavioural and other problems may still be manifest by personality disordered individuals in this treatment, however, and in general clinicians must have a good awareness of the features of the condition. A common mistake is to fail to appreciate when personality disorder is producing mood disturbances, and so to over-diagnose depressive illness. Depressive and anxiety symptoms are among the most commonly encountered in drug misusers, and in cases where antidepressant therapy is clearly indicated, the specific serotonergic re-uptake inhibitors are of particular interest because of their range of possible beneficial effects.

Often the term dual diagnosis is used solely to describe the combination of psychosis and substance misuse, which is a complex area in itself. Many of the drugs of misuse can cause or precipitate psychosis, with stimulants probably being the worst offenders, and opiates, importantly, an exception. The evidence for lasting psychosis produced by drugs, and continuing once drug misuse has stopped, is relatively weak, however, and a number of mechanisms have been described which account for shorter-lived symptoms. A realistic position to adopt is that although demonstrations of causality are inherently difficult, drugs including amphetamines, ecstasy, cocaine, LSD, solvents and cannabis are particularly inadvisable in individuals who have any propensity or vulnerability to psychosis, or an existing psychotic condition, which they may worsen.

Unfortunately, for various reasons to do with typical social situations and cognitive impairments, those with severe mental illness frequently become involved with drug misuse. Studies have shown drug misuse in up to 50% of psychotic individuals, and the rising rates, reflecting drug misuse trends generally, are posing major problems for clinicians providing general psychiatric treatment in the community. Associated drug misuse reduces compliance with treatment and impairs response to psychiatric medications, while dual diagnosis patients have the highest rates of violence, clinical and behavioural problems, and adverse personal circumstances such as homelessness. Unless guarded against, there is a tendency for such patients to drop out of treatment contact, partly because the additional diagnosis may actually exclude them from some elements of either psychiatric or drug misuse services. Liaison between services will not alone solve this problem, but successful treatment is more likely if there are clearly defined roles for each type of service. There may be specially appointed dual diagnosis workers in community teams attached to either general psychiatry or drug misuse, with an emphasis on psychotic patients more likely if referrals come through general psychiatry. Most of the literature on working with dual diagnosis patients comes from ultra-specialist services, with a remit solely for this clinical group. Caseloads in such work need to be small because of the intensive nature of the clinical management required, and so even where there are highly specialized services or workers, most dually diagnosed individuals cannot be directly treated by them. There consequently needs to be an emphasis on training to facilitate better management elsewhere, and principles of managing dual diagnosis patients have been described which would appear to have wide applicability.

# Epilogue

## Future directions

In this book the attempt has been to analyse, in varying degrees of depth, most of the important current issues which pertain to the treatment of drug misuse. In this brief final section we will look ahead, to predict some likely developments, and also the subjects which clinicians will need to particularly address in the short-term future.

### The scope of treatment

In many areas the indicators of drug misuse simply rise steadily, as do those of the various broadly related social trends. We are likely to be faced with increasing demands for treatment services, which although good for job security gives us problems such as lengthy waiting lists. The only potential for a really major impact on these trends would lie in radical measures such as legalization of addictive drugs – extremely unlikely in most of our areas in the foreseeable future – or in enhanced law enforcement. Education and preventive initiatives have their extremely important roles, but in general these are not effective enough to stem the rising tide, while enforcement policies have actually become less severe in recent years, partly because the criminal justice system is also more than full due to the same social trends. Indeed, the courts are increasingly likely to turn to us as on alternative disposal, with the use of formalized treatment orders if necessary.

The direction in which our own drug treatment policies have shifted in recent years has also contributed to the congestion in drug services. The involvement – actual and potential – of drug misusers in the HIV epidemic produced an emphasis on attraction of users into treatment and subsequent retention, and on methadone treatment in general. Although there is an expectation of 'throughput' in methadone services, the treatment has a tendency to become long term even in cases where this was not the original intention, especially when harm-reduction principles are the guiding force. Primary care can be recruited to spread the load of methadone treatment, but any medical service which becomes involved will soon fill its available places, with resultant delays and concerns about access. More clinicians will face debate about prioritization of cases and rationing, especially those of us in publicly-funded health services where competition for funds is intense.

Given these various pressures, we will need to be confident in the effectiveness of our treatments for drug misuse, but also realistic. At the launch of a recent government task force report in the UK on drug services, the soundbite message which was promoted was that 'treatment works'. I have also seen this used in the USA, but surely this claim is only partly sustainable. Some treatments work, some of the time; some treatments work extremely well and easily – detoxification for short-term heroin users, naltrexone, good counselling, and substitution treatments in those who have been dependent for a significant length of time. Other treatments, however, do not work particularly well, such as those for cocaine or amphetamine misuse, and our efforts may not be very productive in individuals in whom drug use is only one of multiple problems. Others tend to recognize this quite well, not least the general public, and so, while investigating and applying the available treatments for different types of drug misuse, we need to form correct judgements about their general effectiveness, in planning services and referral systems. Restricting treatments to those which have a strong evidence base would make case loads more manageable but, as indicated below, it would probably be wrong to apply this in any simple way in drug misuse. After being somewhat neglected in the recent harm-reduction era, the issue of motivation may re-emerge more strongly in the face of overwhelming demand for services.

## Opioid substitution

At present this is the single most important area in drug misuse treatment. Clinicians who witness its almost routine benefits make strong claims that it should be available to all who need it, but once again the demand is such that this is unrealistic in many areas as things stand. We have seen in the review that many of the benefits of substitution treatment are social, notably including reduced crime, and surely calls will increase for it to be funded from sources other than medical or psychiatric budgets. Claims could legitimately be made on crime prevention funding for treatments which have been demonstrated to have that effect, although commentators have suggested that an adequate effect of this kind for some individuals may only be achieved by going beyond standard methadone treatment, to which most of the general evidence relates (e.g. Raistrick 1997).

The advantages and limitations of methadone as a drug will no doubt continue to be debated from various quarters. We have seen that it proves to be an excellent drug in individuals who can adjust to its particular effects, but that that leaves many others who cannot do so. The arguments for giving heroin itself to at least some addicts are seductive, and the trials in Switzerland have received a great deal of attention (Uchtenhagen et al. 1996). In Europe there has been experience with a wide range of substitution drugs, and those in other countries with an interest in flexible treatment look to this if they feel that adherence to a methadone-only policy is too limiting. Unfortunately they do not find much systematic evidence, but at the same time the problems of methadone for a proportion of individuals become ever more apparent as the drug is used more widely, and the arguments for alternatives will become more interesting as studies accumulate.

Two drugs which have been fairly substantially investigated are buprenorphine and levo-alpha-acetyl methadol (LAAM), and the place which these should occupy in treatment will become clearer over the next few years. Buprenorphine is undoubtedly safer (on its own) and less addictive than methadone, and so it will be appealing to use in individuals at risk, and in detoxification. The disparity between a textbook description of a methadone detoxification and the situations which tend to occur in practice is one of the most negative experiences for doctors who attempt to treat drug misusers, and if buprenorphine can increase completion rates in those who are detoxification candidates, this will be greatly welcomed. There are also suggestions that neonatal opiate withdrawal features may be less with buprenorphine than with methadone after treatment in pregnancy, and there are plans for a combination preparation with naloxone to deter injected misuse. LAAM would seem to be indicated for broadly similar patients as methadone, with potential advantages deriving from the less frequent dosing. It may also be possible to gradually increase the intervals between dosing as a stage in a withdrawal process.

## Security of treatment

There is a certain predictability about the debates as to how much security needs to be adopted in methadone treatment, to prevent diversion of supplies and general abuse. Those working in countries with restrictive policies, requiring daily attendance at a treatment centre for supervised consumption of the drug, bemoan the fact that addicts cannot get on with the rest of their lives, whilst those of us in countries with more liberal policies see the problems of trading of medication, overdosage and exploitation of the system. After policies have gone in one direction for a period there is an inevitable swing of the pendulum, while at times the arguments for either approach can seem political just as much as clinical. We must hope that some kind of happy medium can be achieved, as is the case in some services in the UK (we also have the two extremes). Here, it appears that additional restrictions are to be brought in regarding which doctors may prescribe nonstandard treatments, probably including injectable methadone.

If anything, more areas are likely to move towards increasingly secure treatment in the near future, partly because of medico-legal sensitivities. The issue of overdose deaths from treatment drugs weighs particularly heavily and has received much publicity, while also the use of alternative substitution agents will involve stricter controls over dispensing than we have become used to with methadone.

## Evidence-based practice

Clinicians are being exhorted to adopt evidence-based practice (Haynes & Haines 1998), and we are not going to be exempt in drug misuse. Many aspects of this are to be welcomed, if it means that support is more likely to be given to tried and trusted clinical treatments rather than to experimental approaches which are persuasively marketed or seem unduly attractive for some other reason. It is also going to give us problems, however, the most obvious one being that there will be even more danger of over-emphasizing one single treatment approach.

Methadone is very strongly supported by evidence, and indeed is bound to be, given what it is, and the extent to which it has been used. We may argue as to whether it is best seen as a definitive treatment or a so-called heroin substitute, but clearly there are strong elements of the substitution approach, which is hardly used in other forms of drug misuse. If the evidence for effectiveness can include a broad range of social outcomes this will emerge as being in a different league of effectiveness compared with treatments that attempt to withdraw someone from drugs completely, and in some ways the comparison is invalid. There will be narrower arguments between the different substitution treatments in opiate misuse, but any such approach should routinely produce reductions in other drug use, injecting, HIV risk behaviours, and social and financial problems.

A simplistic adherence to the evidence-based principle would mean that we gave methadone to as many heroin addicts as we could, and any other treatments to a lesser degree which reflected the relative strength of the evidence for those. This might be reasonable, but surely at the same time we cannot only be interested in users who have progressed to heroin, and then used that for long enough to become maintenance rather than detoxification candidates, purely because we can use the type of treatment which inevitably has the most impact. If we are in contact with users before they progress to heroin, or are in the early stages of using it, we must attempt treatments for which there is much less supporting evidence, and indeed to some extent we should seek to recruit users in such circumstances.

The aim should be to apply the treatments which have the best supporting evidence relating to the various respective stages of drug misuse, types of drug misuse, and probably types of user within those categories. In doing so we could fall foul of the evidence-based purists, and it is perhaps likely that clinical services will need to identify 'core services', which are strongly evidence-based, and a range of limited other services for drug problems not associated with such established treatments.

In this context it is important to note that the introduction of 'clinical governance' to the substance misuse services should have an impact here. Clinical governance is an essential component of new health service practice (Department of Health 1997) and has been defined as 'a system through which NHS organizations are accountable for continuously improving the quality of their services and safeguarding high standards of care by creating an environment in which excellence in clinical care will flourish' (Scally & Donaldson 1998). It includes professional competence, good use of resources, risk management and patient satisfaction. If this is implemented in the spirit in which it was intended it should have an important impact on services for drug users, and should stimulate a bigger evidence base than that currently occupied mainly by methadone maintenance.

## Stimulant misuse

The search for an effective treatment for cocaine misuse will go on, the latest avenues being a vaccine whereby anticocaine antibodies block the drug's effects (Fox 1997), and the enhancement of enzymatic activity to hasten cocaine excretion (Gorelick 1997). The prospect of any country having a USA-style cocaine and crack epidemic seems to have receded, but many clinicians will see enough of this form of drug misuse to be frustrated by the lack of impact of available treatments. There are often significant subcultural differences between heroin and cocaine scenes in the same localities, and it is increasingly recognized that services need to be tailored in particular ways to attract the cocaine users. Good evidence relating to any treatment or rehabilitative measures will be welcomed, as the transfer from criminal justice system to treatment in particular is difficult if the latter is relatively ineffective, and if there has been violent crime, which seems to be common.

Amphetamine use is often far more widespread, and there will be continued calls for more attention to this problem. The discrepancy between treatment of heroin users and this group has been highlighted now that the subject of amphetamine prescribing has been tentatively broached (Bradbeer et al. 1998). No one believes that this can be anything like as effective as methadone prescribing for opiate misusers overall, but at the same time many clinicians think it unreasonable to discount it out of hand. Considering the commonalities across the forms of drug misuse, it seems illogical that methadone can be so strongly supported and promoted for opiate dependence, while a substitution approach is apparently to be completely denied those dependent on amphetamines. It is to be hoped that the prescribing debate does not unduly dominate the calls for more attention to amphetamine misusers, as various possible treatments of this group, including prescribing, simply need to be moved up the research agenda, given the previous neglect.

## Hepatitis C

Just when everyone was becoming somewhat more relaxed about HIV, with very low prevalences having emerged in many areas, along comes hepatitis C (Coutinho 1998). This is much more infective through blood transmission than HIV (as evidenced by the rates of infection following needlestick injuries), and many services are seeing prevalence rates of 60–70% in drug injectors. The fact that such high rates of transmission have occurred even with the needle exchanges and related initiatives can give ammunition to the critics of harm reduction.

Hepatitis C is a serious disease, with persisting infection in the vast majority of cases, which can lead to cirrhosis and liver carcinoma. Results of treatment with interferon and ribavirin are only moderate, and the forthcoming period will see the liver services develop criteria for treating drug misusers, as evidence on the effects of continued drug use, injecting and other factors emerges. It seems that alcohol use adversely affects prognosis, while treatment is more effective if started early, and so drug services will need to become used to testing and advising patients appropriately. Whereas only some areas have been faced with large numbers of drug misusers becoming ill with HIV and AIDS, it will be hepatitis C that represents the main medical illness affecting patients in our clinics, to the extent of early fatality in many cases.

## Detoxification

A widespread development in the UK in the last few years has been detoxification using lofexidine, particularly for young, early-stage heroin users. Services have found this an excellent addition to the treatment options, given the rapidly rising numbers of such individuals presenting. Evidence for the direct effectiveness of lofexidine is accumulating, while also it may be observed that this medication has provided the vehicle for drug teams to carry out intensively-supported home detoxifications, after a period in which the focus was overwhelmingly on methadone maintenance. Many good protocols have been developed by individual services, and the experience of teams that do a lot of this work should be instructive for those who find it more difficult to adopt the assertive tactics which are required.

This development has been popular with users who have no wish to take methadone, as has the availability of naltrexone after detoxification. The place of naltrexone within treatment should become more firmly established, and it will be important to see whether a depot preparation is feasible. Naltrexone is generally given to well motivated patients, but inevitably some supplies of tablets are diverted, and the situations in which abuse occurs will need clarification, so that they can be guarded against.

## Child protection

It is fair to say that as treatment became much more open and accessible on harm-reduction principles at the time when HIV prevention was being emphasized, there was a tendency to underplay the effects which drug misuse may have on users' children. It was recognized that one of the reasons why women tended to be under-represented in treatment services was because they had particular concerns that there would be statutory involvement with their children, and in generally encouraging users to come forward there was much reassurance that this was not going to be the case. There is now a definite growing realization that some of the outcomes in children of drug misusers – including patients on methadone – can be very poor, in terms of injuries, various forms of neglect, noncompliance with paediatric surveillance, and subsequent education failure and antisocial behaviours. There are no doubt many important associations within such relationships, and recent studies have investigated direct effects of substance use in pregnancy, psychological deficits in children of users and possible transmission factors, as well as situations of child abuse and neglect (Wolstein et al. 1998). The last type of study tends to appear in the child abuse literature (e.g. Jaudes et al. 1995, Wolock & Magura 1996), and so drug workers may not be aware of them, but there must be better general appreciation of the problems of children in our work with the parents. The particular sensitivities in this area are all too obvious, but explicit assessments of child care must be included if it is to be established which treatments genuinely help in this area, alongside other treatment benefits.

# Appendix 1

## Protocols for quick detoxification from heroin

These protocols relate to treatment as described on pages 84–87. This is the form in which information is given to patients, except for the additional notes.

### Method 1 – Symptomatic medication

These medications are to be taken only if required

**Diazepam (5 mg tablets) (reduces muscle cramps, anxiety and cravings)**
Take tablets one or two at a time, with at least four hours between doses.
*Maximum* daily dose:

| Day | No. of tablets |
| --- | --- |
| 1 | 2 |
| 2 | 4 |
| 3 | 6 |
| 4 | 6 |
| 5 | 4 |
| 6 | 2 |
| 7 | 1 |
| Total | 25 tablets |

**Nitrazepam (5 mg tablets) (helps sleep)**
Unfortunately sleep may be poor even with these sleeping tablets. Do not take more than the recommended dose, as this can be dangerous and is unlikely to be effective.
*Maximum* dose – two tablets at night. Total 14 tablets.

**Buscopan (10 mg tablets) (reduces stomach spasm)**
Take tablets two at a time, with at least four hours between doses
*Maximum* dose – eight tablets in 24 hours. Total 30 tablets.

**Lomotil (2.5 mg tablets) (reduces diarrhoea)**
Ensure plenty of fluids are taken during any periods of diarrhoea
and/or vomiting.
Take four tablets initially, when diarrhoea starts, then two tablets
every six hours until it stops.
Total 30 tablets.

Note: To avoid over-use of medication and to facilitate contact, the total
medication supply may be divided into two prescriptions, with the
worker providing the second one two to three days into the detoxification.

## Method 2 – Lofexidine plus symptomatic medication

All medications are to be taken only if required

**Lofexidine (0.2 mg tablets) (treatment for withdrawal symptoms)**
Take tablets at regular intervals, as shown. The following are the
*maximum* doses. Remember to check your pulse before each dose and
take the medication only if it is above 60 beats/minute.

|         | 9:00 am | 1:00 pm | 5:00 pm | 9:00 pm | Total tablets in 24 hours |
|---------|---------|---------|---------|---------|---------------------------|
| Day 1   | 2       | 2       | 2       | 2       | 8                         |
| Day 2   | 3       | 2       | 2       | 3       | 10                        |
| Day 3   | 3       | 3       | 3       | 3       | 12                        |
| Day 4   | 3       | 3       | 3       | 3       | 12                        |
| Day 5   | 3       | 2       | 2       | 3       | 10                        |
| Day 6   | 2       | 2       | 2       | 2       | 8                         |
| Day 7   | —       | —       | —       | —       | 0                         |

*Diazepam, nitrazepam, Buscopan and Lomotil* – as in Method 1.
Notes: The lofexidine and symptomatic medication courses run concur-
rently. As with Method 1, the total supply may be divided into two
prescriptions.

## Method 3 – Dihydrocodeine plus symptomatic medication

Dihydrocodeine (30 mg tablets)
Take medication in divided doses four times a day, with four to six hours between doses. The following are the *maximum* daily doses.

| Day | No. of tablets |
|---|---|
| 1 | 12 |
| 2 | 18 |
| 3 | 20 |
| 4 | 20 |
| 5 | 20 |
| 6 | 18 |
| 7 | 16 |
| may start here, see note | |
| 8 | 14 |
| 9 | 12 |
| 10 | 10 |
| start symptomatic medication here | |
| 11 | 8 |
| 12 | 6 |
| 13 | 4 |
| 14 | 2 |

*Diazepam, nitrazepam, Buscopan and Lomotil* – as in Method 1.

Notes: In this method the medication supply is always divided into a series of prescriptions, each for three to four days' supply.

The symptomatic medication only begins four days from the end of the dihydrocodeine course, as indicated.

Not all patients require the relatively high dihydrocodeine doses suggested at the start of the course. If this method is used to detoxify from low levels of heroin, a shorter course may be used, as indicated. Some adjustments may be necessary to have the maximum dihydrocodeine dose about three days into the detoxification.

# Appendix 2

## Opioid equivalent dosages

Knowledge of equivalent dosages is required when methadone substitution treatment is initiated, or when a patient is changed from methadone to an alternative opioid. The following is a guide to the *pharmacological equivalents* of opioids compared to methadone, but it must be emphasized that daily dosages *in practice* may not be in the same ratios. This is because drug half-lives must also be taken into account, so that *relatively higher dosages than indicated are required of shorter-acting drugs* – including diamorphine, morphine and dihydrocodeine – where repeated dosing in a day is needed.

| Drug | Dose | Methadone equivalent |
| --- | --- | --- |
| Diamorphine | 10 mg | 10 mg |
| 'Street' heroin | 1 g of powder | 50–60 mg * |
| Morphine | 10 mg | 10 mg |
| Dipipanone | 10 mg | 4 mg |
| Dihydrocodeine | 30 mg | 3 mg |
| Dextromoramide | 10 mg | 10–20 mg |
| Pethidine | 50 mg | 5 mg |
| Buprenorphine | 0.2 mg | 5 mg |
| Pentazocine | 50 mg | 4 mg |
| Codeine phosphate | 30 mg | 2 mg |

Based on Department of Health (1991)
* This is what is usually required clinically, given purity of street heroin of about 20–30%

# Glossary

This explains some of the terms which are used in the book. Drugs slang is not included, as this varies greatly between countries and local areas.

**Addictiveness**    Propensity of a drug to cause dependence, particularly withdrawal symptoms

**Agonist**    A drug which produces a specified chemical action

**Amphetamine**    Stimulant drug, usually in the form of a very impure powder

**Ampoule**    Glass phial of a pharmaceutical drug

**Antagonist**    A drug which produces the opposite of a specified chemical action

**Barbiturates**    Tranquillizers commonly used before the benzodiazepines were introduced – Tuinal, Seconal, etc

**Benzodiazepines**    Widely prescribed tranquillizers – diazepam, nitrazepam, etc

**Buprenorphine**    Medication with both opioid agonist and antagonist actions

**Cannabis**    Herbal sedative drug, with various forms derived from different parts of the plant

**Cocaine**    Stimulant drug, has typically been relatively expensive. The powder form is cocaine hydrochloride, but increasingly the more potent *crack* is used, in the form of crystalline 'rocks'

**Community treatment**    Treatment in which individuals are managed in or near their own home, often in liaison with other local agencies

**Cyclizine**    Antiemetic medication, tablets of which are abused by injection

**Dependence**    State in which there is a strong requirement for a drug, particularly characterized by varying degrees of tolerance, craving and withdrawal symptoms. If withdrawal symptoms are of a bodily kind, e.g. tremor or fits, the term *physical dependence* can be used

**Detoxification**    The process of controlled withdrawal from a drug

**Dextromoramide** (Palfium)    Opioid medication, frequently abused by injection

**Diamorphine** Heroin – the chemical term diamorphine may be used to refer to the pharmaceutical preparation

**Dipipanone** (Diconal) Opioid medication, highly regarded by drug misusers

**Dual diagnosis** Strictly speaking, refers to any combination of psychiatric (or other) diagnoses, but increasingly used to indicate substance misuse plus a psychiatric condition, e.g. schizophrenia, depression

**Ecstasy** Methylenedioxymethamphetamine – a stimulant drug with additional semihallucinogenic effects

**Hard drugs** A term usually discouraged by professionals, but which can be used to refer to the more addictive drugs

**Harm reduction** A range of policy measures aimed at reducing the harm which comes from drug misuse, rather than eliminating it completely

**Heroin** Highly addictive sedative drug, usually in the form of an impure powder

**HIV** Human Immunodeficiency Virus, which exists in different forms. Also refers to the fatal disease caused by the virus, AIDS

**HIV risk behaviours** Behaviours which increase the risk of acquiring or transmitting HIV, including various injecting and sexual practices

**Illicit drugs** Drugs which are illegal to obtain or use in a specific country

**Injectable medication** Usually refers to preparations which are meant to be injected, e.g. methadone ampoules, although can refer to tablets, etc., which may be abused by injection

**LAAM** Levo-alpha-acetyl methadol. A long-acting equivalent of methadone

**Lofexidine** Analogue of clonidine with fewer adverse effects, used in opiate detoxification

**Low threshold treatment** Treatment – usually methadone – made easy to obtain, as part of a harm-reduction approach

**Maintenance** Ongoing substitution treatment, usually with methadone

**MDMA** Methylenedioxymethamphetamine. See ecstasy

**Methadone** Synthetic opioid medication used as the so-called 'heroin substitute'

**Motivation** Desire to change drug-taking behaviour or have treatment. May be enhanced by *motivational interviewing*

**Naltrexone** Opioid antagonist used to block the effects of heroin or related drugs

**Narcotic**   Technically means sleep-inducing, but various usages refer to opiates or 'hard drugs' in general

**Narcotic blockade**   Effect by which methadone is claimed to nullify the actions of other opiates or opioids if taken

**Opiates**   Naturally occurring heroin-like drugs, including heroin itself

**Opioids**   Synthetic heroin-like drugs

**Palfium**   See dextromoromide

**Primary care**   The general practice treatment setting

**Recreational drug use**   A much derided term which refers to drug use which is relatively unproblematic and seen as a lifestyle choice

**Rehabilitation**   The process of learning to live without drugs. May be formally approached in a residential *rehabilitation centre*. A broader usage of the term refers to almost any treatment

**Secondary service**   Specialist service to which general practitioners and others may refer

**Sedative drugs** ('downers')   Range of drugs with predominantly sedating and tranquillizing effects

**Serotonin**   Brain chemical which is important in determining mood and some of the effects of drugs. One group of antidepressants is the *specific serotonergic re-uptake inhibitors*

**Soft drugs**   See reference to hard drugs. In this distinction, soft drugs are the less addictive kinds

**Solvent misuse**   Problematic use, by sniffing, of glues, lighter fuels, etc which contain various volatile substances

**Stimulant drugs** ('uppers')   Range of drugs with predominantly stimulant and energizing effects

**Substance misuse**   Problematic use of any chemical substance

**Substitution treatment**   Treatment in which an individual receives a medication with broadly similar effects to their drug of dependence

**Therapeutic community**   Residential rehabilitation centre based on a particularly strong 'concept' or religious theme

**Tolerance**   The phenomenon whereby increasing amounts of drug are required to achieve the same effect

**Twelve-step treatment**   The conceptual basis of the methods adopted by Alcoholics Anonymous, Narcotics Anonymous and related organizations. It is considered that 'recovery' from addiction is achieved by addressing 12 specified steps in turn

**Volatile substances**   See solvent misuse

**Withdrawal**   This term is used to refer both to the symptoms which occur on stopping a drug and to the process of detoxification

# References

Abed RT & Neira-Munoz E (1990). A survey of general practitioners' opinion and attitude to drug addicts and addiction. *British Journal of Addiction*, **85**, 131–6

Abraham HD & Aldridge AM (1993). Adverse consequences of lysergic acid diethylamide. *Addiction*, **88**, 1327–34

Advisory Council on the Misuse of Drugs (1982). *Treatment and Rehabilitation*. Department of Health, Her Majesty's Stationery Office, London

Advisory Council on the Misuse of Drugs (1988). *AIDS and Drug Misuse, Part 1*. Department of Health, Her Majesty's Stationery Office, London

Advisory Council on the Misuse of Drugs (1989). *AIDS and Drug Misuse, Part 2*. Department of Health, Her Majesty's Stationery Office, London

Advisory Council on the Misuse of Drugs (1993). *AIDS and Drug Misuse Update*. Department of Health, Her Majesty's Stationery Office, London

Advisory Council on the Misuse of Drugs (1995). *Volatile Substance Abuse*. Department of Health, Her Majesty's Stationery Office, London

Amass L, Bickel WK, Higgins ST & Badger GJ (1994). Alternate-day dosing during buprenorphine treatment of opioid dependence. *Life Sciences*, **54**, 1215–28

American Psychiatric Association (1994). Position statement on methadone maintenance treatment. *American Journal of Psychiatry*, **151**, 792–4

Andreasson S, Allebeck P, Engstrom A et al. (1987). Cannabis and schizophrenia. A longitudinal study of Swedish conscripts. *The Lancet*, **ii**, 1483–6

Arndt IO, McLellan AT, Dorozynsky L, Woody GE & O'Brien CP (1994). Desipramine treatment for cocaine dependence: role of antisocial personality disorder. *Journal of Nervous and Mental Disease*, **182**, 151–6

Babor TF & Grant M (1989). From clinical research to secondary prevention: international collaboration in the development of the Alcohol Use Disorders Identification Test (AUDIT). *Alcohol Health and Research World*, **13**, 371–4

Bailey LG, Maxwell S & Brandabur MM (1997). Substance abuse as a risk factor for tardive dyskinesia: a retrospective analysis of 1,027 patients. *Psychopharmacological Bulletin*, **33**, 177–81

Ball JC & Ross A (1991). *The Effectiveness of Methadone Maintenance Treatment: Patients, Programs, Services and Outcome*. New York: Springer-Verlag

Ball JC & van de Wijngaart GF (1994). A Dutch addict's view of methadone maintenance – an American and a Dutch appraisal. *Addiction*, **89**, 799–802

Bartels SJ & Drake RE (1996). A pilot study of residential treatment for dual diagnoses. *Journal of Nervous and Mental Disease*, **184**, 379–81

Bartels SJ, Drake RE, Wallach MA et al. (1991). Characteristic hostility in schizophrenic outpatients. *Schizophrenia Bulletin*, **17**, 163–71

Bartels SJ, Teague GB, Drake RE et al. (1993). Service utilization and costs associated with substance use disorder among severely mentally ill patients. *Journal of Nervous and Mental Disease*, **181**, 227–32

Bartter T & Gooberman LL (1996). Rapid opiate detoxification. *American Journal of Drug & Alcohol Abuse*, **22**, 489–95

Battersby M, Farrell M, Gossop M, Robson P & Strang J (1992). 'Horse trading': prescribing injectable opiates to opiate addicts. A descriptive study. *Drug and Alcohol Review*, **11**, 35–42

Bearn J, Gossop M & Strang J (1996). Randomised double-blind comparison of lofexidine and methadone in the inpatient treatment of opiate withdrawal. *Drug and Alcohol Dependence*, **43**, 87–91

Beel A, Maycock B & McLean N (1998). Current perspectives on anabolic steroids. *Drug and Alcohol Review*, **17**, 87–103

Bell J, Fernandes D & Batey R (1990a). Heroin users seeking methadone treatment. *Medical Journal of Australia*, **152**, 361–4

Bell J, Bowron P, Lewis J & Batey R (1990b). Serum levels of methadone in maintenance clients who persist in illicit drug use. *British Journal of Addiction*, **85**, 1599–602

Benowitz NL (1992). Clinical pharmacology and toxicology of cocaine. *Pharmacology and Toxicology*, **72**, 3–12

Bentley AJ & Busuttil A (1996). Deaths among drug abusers in south-east Scotland (1989–1994). *Medicine, Science & The Law*, **36**, 231–6

Bertschy G (1995). Methadone maintenance treatment: an update. *European Archives of Psychiatry and Clinical Neuroscience*, **245**, 114–24

Bickel WK & Amass L (1995). Buprenorphine treatment of opioid dependence: a review. *Experimental and Clinical Psychopharmacology*, **3**, 477–89

Bickel WK, Stitzer ML, Bigelow GE, Liebson IA, Jasinski DR & Johnson RE (1988). A clinical trial of buprenorphine: comparison with methadone in the detoxification of heroin addicts. *Clinical Pharmacology and Therapeutics*, **43**, 72–8

Bigwood CS & Coehelho AJ (1990). Methadone and caries. *British Dental Journal*, **168**, 231

Bond A (1993). The risks of taking benzodiazepines. In: Hallstrom, C (ed.) *Benzodiazepine Dependence*. Oxford: Oxford Medical Publications, pp. 34–45

Boutros NN & Bowers MB Jnr (1996). Chronic substance-induced psychotic disorders: state of the literature. *Journal of Neuropsychiatry and Clinical Neuroscience*, **8**, 262–9

Boys A, Lenton S & Norcross K (1997). Polydrug use at raves by a Western Australian sample. *Drug and Alcohol Review*, **16**, 227–34

Bradbeer TM, Fleming PM, Charlton P & Crichton JS (1998). Survey of amphetamine prescribing in England and Wales. *Drug and Alcohol Review*, **17**, 299–304

Brahen LS & Brewer C (1993). Naltrexone in the criminal justice system. In: Brewer, C (ed.) *Treatment Options in Addiction*. London: Gaskell, pp. 46–53

Brewer C (1993). Naltrexone on the prevention of relapse and opiate detoxification. In: Brewer, C (ed.) *Treatment Options in Addiction*, London: Gaskell, pp. 54–62

Brewer C (1996). On the specific effectiveness, and under-valuing, of pharmacological treatments for addiction: a comparison of methadone, naltrexone and disulfiram with psychosocial interventions. *Addiction Research*, **3**, 297–313

Brewer C (1997). Ultra-rapid, antagonist-precipitated opiate detoxification under general anaesthesia or sedation. *Addiction Biology*, **2**, 291–302

Brooner RK, Greenfield L, Schmidt C & Bigelow GE (1993). Antisocial personality disorder and HIV infection among intravenous drug abusers. *American Journal of*

*Psychiatry*, **150**, 53–8

Brunette MF & Drake RE (1997). Gender differences in patients with schizophrenia and substance abuse. *Comprehensive Psychiatry*, **38**, 109–16

Budney AJ, Bickel WK & Amass L (1998). Marijuana use and treatment outcome among opioid-dependent patients. *Addiction*, **93**, 493–503

Buning EC, van Brussel GHA, van Santen MD & van Santen G (1990). The 'methadone by bus' project in Amsterdam. *British Journal of Addiction*, **85**, 1247–50

Capelhorn JRM (1994). A comparison of abstinence-oriented and indefinite methadone maintenance treatment. *International Journal of the Addictions*, **29**, 1361–75

Capelhorn JRM (1998). Deaths in the first two weeks of maintenance treatment in NSW in 1994: identifying cases of iatrogenic methadone toxicity. *Drug and Alcohol Review*, **17**, 9–17

Capelhorn JRM & Bell J (1991). Methadone dosage and retention of patients in maintenance treatment. *Medical Journal of Australia*, **154**, 195–9

Capelhorn JRM, Bell J, Kleinbaum DG & Gebski VJ (1993). Methadone dose and heroin use during maintenance treatment. *Addiction*, **88**, 119–24

Capelhorn JRM, Dalton MSYN, Cluff MC & Petrenas AM (1994). Retention in methadone maintenance and heroin addicts' risk of death. *Addiction*, **89**, 203–7

Capelhorn JRM & Ross MW (1995). Methadone maintenance and the likelihood of risky needle-sharing. *International Journal of the Addictions*, **30**, 685–98

Chaisson RE, Bacchetti P, Osmond D, Brodie B, Sande MA & Moss AR (1989). Cocaine use and HIV infection in intravenous drug users in San Francisco. *Journal of the American Medical Association*, **261**, 561–5

Chapleo CB & Walter DS (1997). The buprenorphine–naloxone combination product. *Research and Clinical Forums*, **19**, 55–8

Chapleo CB, Reisinger M & Rindom H (1997). European update. *Research and Clinical Forums*, **19**, 33–8

Cheskin LJ, Fudala PJ & Johnson RE (1994). A controlled comparison of buprenorphine and clonidine for acute detoxification from opioids. *Drug and Alcohol Dependence*, **36**, 115–21

Chick J (1996). Medication in the treatment of alcohol dependence. *Advances in Psychiatric Treatment*, **2**, 249–57

Chick J, Ritson B, Connaughton J, Stewart A & Chick J (1988). Advice versus extended treatment for alcoholism: a controlled study. *British Journal of Addiction*, **83**, 159–70

Chowdhury JR & Bhattacharjee D (1995). General practitioners and changing scenario in drug abuse. *Journal of the Indian Medical Association*, **93**, 155–6

Cinciripini PM, Lapitsky L Seay S, Wallfisch A, Kitchens K & Van Vunkis H (1995). The effects of smoking schedules on cessation outcome: can we improve on common methods of gradual and abrupt nicotine withdrawal? *Journal of Consulting and Clinical Psychology*, **63**, 388–99

Clark JC, Milroy CM & Forrest ARW (1995). Deaths from methadone use. *Journal of Clinical Forensic Medicine*, **2**, 143–4

Connell PH (1958). *Amphetamine Psychosis*. Institute of Psychiatry Maudsley Monograph No. 5. London; Oxford University Press

Cook CH (1988). The Minnesota model in the management of drug and alcohol dependency: miracle, method or myth? Part I: The philosophy and the programme. *British Journal of Addiction*, **83**, 625–34

Corcoran JP & Longo ED (1992). Psychological treatment of anabolic–androgenic steroid-dependent individuals. *Journal of Substance Abuse Treatment*, **9**, 229–35

Coutinho RA (1998). HIV and hepatitis C among injecting drug users. *British Medical Journal*, **317**, 424–5

Covi L, Hess JM, Kreiter NA & Haertzen CA (1995). Effects of combined fluoxetine and counselling in the outpatient treatment of cocaine abusers. *American Journal of Drug & Alcohol Abuse*, **21**, 327–44

Craig RJ, Olson R & Shalton G (1990). Improvement in psychological functioning among drug abusers: inpatient treatment compared to outpatient methadone maintenance. *Journal of Substance Abuse Treatment*, **7**, 11–19

Cregler L & Mark H (1986). Medical complications of cocaine abuse. *New England Journal of Medicine*, **315**, 1495–500

Crofts N, Nigro L, Oman K, Stevenson G & Sherman J (1997). Methadone maintenance and hepatitis C virus infection among injecting drug users. *Addiction*, **92**, 999–1005

Cuffel BJ, Shumway M, Chouljian TL et al. (1994). A longitudinal study of substance use and community violence in schizophrenia. *Journal of Nervous and Mental Disease*, **182**, 704–8

Darke S (1994). Benzodiazepine use among injecting users, problems and implications. *Addiction*, **89**, 379–82

Darke S (1998). The effectiveness of methadone maintenance treatment. 3: Moderators of treatment outcome. In: Ward J, Mattick RP, Hall W (eds.) *Methadone Maintenance Treatment and Other Opioid Replacement Therapies*, London: Harwood, pp. 75–90

Darke S, Hall W & Carless J (1990). Drug use, injecting practices and sexual behaviour of opioid users in Sydney, Australia. *British Journal of Addiction*, **85**, 1603–9

Darke S, Hall W, Wodak A, Heather N & Ward J (1992a). Development and validation of a multi-dimensional instrument for assessing outcome of treatment among opiate users: the Opiate Treatment Index. *British Journal of Addiction*, **87**, 733–42

Darke S, Hall W, Ross MW & Wodak A (1992b). Benzodiazepine use and HIV risk-taking behaviour among injecting drug users. *Drug and Alcohol Dependence*, **31**, 31–6

Darke S, Swift W, Hall W & Ross M (1993). Drug use, HIV risk-taking and psychosocial correlates of benzodiazepine use among methadone maintenance clients. *Drug and Alcohol Dependence*, **34**, 67–70

Darke S, Ross J & Cohen J (1994a). The use of benzodiazepines among regular amphetamine users. *Addiction*, **89**, 1683–90

Darke S, Hall W & Swift W (1994b). Prevalence, symptoms and correlates of antisocial personality disorder among methadone maintenance clients. *Drug and Alcohol Dependence*, **34**, 253–7

Darke S, Swift W & Hall W (1994c). Prevalence, severity and correlates of psychological morbidity among methadone maintenance clients. *Addiction*, **89**, 211–17

Darke S, Ross J & Hall W (1996a). Overdose among heroin users in Sydney, Australia. I. Prevalence and correlates of non-fatal overdose. *Addiction*, **91**, 405–11

Darke S, Ross J & Hall W (1996b). Overdose among heroin users in Sydney, Australia. II. Responses to overdose. *Addiction*, **91**, 413–17

Darke S & Zador D (1996). Fatal heroin overdose: a review. *Addiction*, **91**, 1765–72

Darke S, Sunjic S, Zador & Prolov T (1997). A comparison of blood toxicology of heroin-related deaths and current heroin users in Sydney, Australia. *Drug and Alcohol Dependence*, **47**, 45–53

Davies A & Huxley P (1997). Survey of general practitioners' opinions on treatment of opiate users. *British Medical Journal*, **314**, 1173–4

Davoli M, Perucci CA, Forastiere F, Doyle P, Rapiti E, Zaccarelli M et al. (1993). Risk factors for overdose mortality: a case control study within a cohort of intravenous drug users. *International Journal of Epidemiology*, **22**, 273–7

Davoli M, Perucci CA, Rapiti E, Bargagli AM, D'Ippoliti D, Forastiere F & Abeni D (1997). A persistent rise in mortality among injection drug users in Rome, 1980 through 1992. *American Journal of Public Health*, **87**, 851–3

Dawe S, Griffiths P, Gossop M & Strang J (1991). Should opiate addicts be involved in controlling their own detoxification? A comparison of fixed versus negotiable schedules. *British Journal of Addiction*, **86**, 977–82

Deehan A, Taylor C & Strang J (1997). The general practitioner, the drug misuser, and the alcohol misuser: major differences in general practitioner activity, therapeutic commitment, and 'shared care' proposals. *British Journal of General Practice*, **47**, 705–9

De Leon G, Staines GL & Sacks S (1997). Passages: a therapeutic community oriented day treatment model for methadone maintained clients. *Journal of Drug Issues*, **27**, 341–66

Department of Health (1991). *Drug Misuse and Dependence: Guidelines on Clinical Management*. London: HMSO

Department of Health (1997). *The New NHS*. London: HMSO

Doberczak TM, Kandall SR & Friedmann P (1993). Relationships between maternal methadone dosage, maternal-neonatal methadone levels, and neonatal withdrawal. *Obstetrics and Gynaecology*, **81**, 936–40

Dole VP (1973). Detoxification of methadone patients and public policy. *Journal of the American Medical Association*, **226**, 747–52

Dole VP (1988). Implications of methadone maintenance for theories of narcotic addiction. *Journal of the American Medical Association*, **260**, 3025–9

Dole VP & Nyswander M (1965). A medical treatment for diacetylmorphine (heroin) addiction. *Journal of the American Medical Association*, **193**, 80–84

Dole VP, Nyswander M & Kreek MJ (1966). Narcotic blockade. *Archives of Internal Medicine*, **118**, 304–9

Dole VP, Robinson JW, Orraca J, Towns E, Searcy P & Caine E (1969). Methadone treatment of randomly selected criminal addicts. *New England Journal of Medicine*, **280**, 1372–5

Dolovich LR, Addis A, Vaillancourt JMR, Power JDB, Koren G & Einarson TR (1998). Benzodiazepine use in pregnancy and major malformations or oral cleft: meta-analysis of cohort and case-control studies. *British Medical Journal*, **317**, 839–43

Donmall M, Seivewright NA, Douglas J, Draycott T & Millar T (1995). *The National Cocaine Treatment Study*. Report to Department of Health, London

Drake RE & Wallach MA (1989). Substance abuse among the chronically mentally ill. *Hospital and Community Psychiatry*, **40**, 1041–6

Drake RE, Bartels SJ, Teagues GB, Noordsy DL & Clark RE (1993). Treatment of substance abuse in severely mentally ill patients. *Journal of Nervous and Mental Disease*, **181**, 606–11

Drake RE, Mueser KT, Clark RE et al. (1996). The course, treatment and outcome of substance disorder in persons with severe mental illness. *American Journal of Orthopsychiatry*, **66**, 42–51

Drummer OH, Opeskin K, Syrjanen M & Cordner SM (1992). Methadone toxicity causing death in 10 subjects starting on a methadone maintenance program. *American Journal of Medicine and Pathology*, **13**, 346–50

Drummond DC, Turkington D, Rahman MZ, Mullin PJ & Jackson P (1989). Chlordiazepoxide versus methadone in opiate withdrawal: a preliminary double blind trial. *Drug and Alcohol Dependence*, **23**, 63–71

Duszynski DR, Nieto FJ & Valente CM (1995). Reported practices, attitudes, and confidence levels of primary care physicians regarding patients who abuse alcohol and other drugs. *Maryland Medical Journal*, **44**, 439–46

Edwards G & Gross MM (1976). Alcohol dependence: provisional description of a clinical syndrome. *British Medical Journal*, **1**, 1058–61

Edwards G, Orford J, Egert S, Guthrie S, Hawker A, Hensman C, Mitcheson M, Oppenheimer E & Taylor C (1977). Alcoholism: a controlled trial of 'treatment' and 'advice'. *Journal of Studies on Alcohol*, **38**, 1004–31

Edwards G, Marshall EJ & Cook CCH (1997). *The Treatment of Drinking Problems: A Guide for the Helping Professions*. Cambridge: Cambridge University Press

Eissenberg T, Bigelow GE, Strain EC, Walsh SL, Brooner RK, Stitzer ML & Johnson RE (1997). Dose-related efficacy of levomethadyl acetate for treatment of opioid dependence. *Journal of the American Medical Association*, **277**, 1945–51

Eklund C, Melin L, Hiltunen & Borg S (1994). Detoxification from methadone maintenance treatment in Sweden: long-term outcome and effects on quality of life and life situation. *The International Journal of the Addictions*, **29**, 627–45

Eveleigh B (1995). The use of lofexidine in an outpatient methadone detoxification programme. *International Journal of Drug Policy*, **6**, 2–3

Farrell M, Battersby M & Strang J (1990). Screening for hepatitis B and vaccination of injecting drug users in NHS drug treatment services. *British Journal of Addiction*, **85**, 1657–9

Farrell M, Ward J, Mattick R, Hall W, Stimson GV, des Jarlais D, Gossop M & Strang J (1994). Methadone maintenance treatment in opiate dependence: a review. *British Medical Journal*, **309**, 997–1001

Farrell M, Neeleman J, Gossop M, Griffiths P, Buning E, Finch E & Strang J (1995). Methadone provision in the European Union. *International Journal of Drug Policy*, **6**, 168–72

Farrell M, Neeleman, J, Griffiths P & Strang J (1996). Suicide and overdose among opiate addicts. *Addiction*, **91**, 321–3

Farren CK (1997). The use of naltrexone, an opiate antagonist, in the treatment of opiate addiction. *Irish Journal of Psychological Medicine*, **14**, 26–31

Federman EB, Costello EJ, Angold A, Farmer EMZ, Erkanli A (1997). Development of substance use and psychiatric comorbidity in an epidemiologic study of white and American Indian young adolescents. The Great Smoky Mountains Study. *Drug and Alcohol Dependence*, **44**, 69–78

Fiore MC, Smith SS, Jorenby DE & Baker TB (1994). The effectiveness of the nicotine patch for smoking cessation: a meta-analysis. *Journal of the American Medical Association*, **271**, 1940–7

Fischer C, Hatzidimitrious G, Wlos J, Katz J & Ricaurte G (1995). Reorganization of ascending 5–HT axon projections in animals previously exposed to the recreational drug ( ±)3,4–methylenedioxymethamphetamine (MDMA, 'Ecstasy'). *The Journal of Neuroscience*, **15**, 5476–85

Fischer G, Presslich O, Diamant K, Schneider C, Pezawas L & Kasper S (1996). Oral morphine-sulphate in the treatment of opiate dependent patients. *Alcoholism*, **32**, 35–43

Flanagan RJ & Ives RJ (1994). Volatile substance abuse. *Bulletin on Narcotics*, **46**, 49–78

Flaum M & Schultz SK (1996). When does amphetamine-induced psychosis become schizophrenia? *American Journal of Psychiatry*, **153**, 812–15

Fleming PM & Roberts D (1994). Is the prescription of amphetamine justified as a harm reduction measure? *Journal of the Royal Society of Health*, June, 127–30

Foltin RW & Fischman MW (1996). Effects of methadone or buprenorphine maintenance on the subjective and reinforcing effects of intravenous cocaine in humans. *Journal of Pharmacology and Experimental Therapeutics*, **278**, 1153–64

Fox BS (1997). Development of a therapeutic vaccine for the treatment of cocaine addiction. *Drug and Alcohol Dependence*, **48**, 153–8

Franke DL, Leistikow BN, Offord KP, Schmidt L & Hurt RD (1995). Physician referrals for smoking cessation: outcome in those who show and don't show. *Preventive Medicine*, **24**, 194–200

Frischer M, Bloor M, Goldberg D, Clark J, Green S & McKeganey N (1993). Mortality among injecting drug users: a critical reappraisal. *Journal of Epidemiology and Community Health*, **47**, 59–63

Frischer M, Goldberg D, Rahman M & Berney L (1997). Mortality and survival among a cohort of drug injectors in Glasgow, 1982–1994. *Addiction*, **92**, 419–27

Fugelstadt A, Rajis J, Bottiger M & Gerhardsson de Verdier M (1995). Mortality among HIV-infected intravenous drug addicts in Stockholm in relation to methadone treatment. *Addiction*, **90**, 711–16

Fugelstadt A, Annell A, Rajis J & Agren G (1997). Mortality and causes and manner of death among drug addicts in Stockholm during the period 1981–1992. *Acta Psychiatrica Scandinavica*, **96**, 169–75

Galanter M, Egelko S, De Leon G, Rohrs C & Franco H (1992). Crack cocaine abusers in the general hospital: assessment and initiation of care. *American Journal of Psychiatry*, **149**, 810–15

Galanter M, Egelko S, Edwards H & Vergaray M (1994). A treatment system for combined psychiatric and addictive illness. *Addiction*, **89**, 1227–35

Gawin FH & Kleber HD (1986). Abstinence symptomatology and psychiatric diagnoses in cocaine abusers: clinical observations. *Archives of General Psychiatry*, **43**, 107–13

Gearing MF (1977). Methadone maintenance in the treatment of heroin addicts in New York City: a ten year review. In: Roisin L, Shiraki H & Grcevic N (eds). *Neurotoxicology*, Vol. 1. New York: Raven Press, pp. 71–9.

Gerra G, Marcato A, Caccavari R et al. (1995). Clonidine and opiate receptor antagonists in the treatment of heroin addiction. *Journal of Substance Abuse Treatment*, **12**, 35–41.

Ghodse AH & Kreek MJ (1997). A rave at ecstasy. *Current Opinion in Psychiatry*, **10**, 191–3

Giannini AJ, Miller NS, Loiselle RH & Turner CE (1993). Cocaine-associated violence and relationship to route of administration. *Journal of Substance Abuse Treatment*, **10**, 67–9

Gibb DM, MacDonagh SE, Gupta R, Tookey PA, Peckham CS & Ades AE (1998). Factors affecting uptake of antenatal HIV testing in London: results of a multi-centre study. *British Medical Journal*, **316**, 259–62

Gill K, Nolimal D & Crowley TJ (1992). Antisocial personality disorder, HIV risk behaviour and retention in methadone maintenance therapy. *Drug and Alcohol Dependence*, **30**, 247–52

Glanz A (1986). Findings of a national survey of the role of general practitioners in the treatment of opiate misuse: dealing with the opiate misuser. *British Medical Journal*, **293**, 486–8

Goedert JJ, Pizza G, Gritti FM, Costigliola P, Boschini A, Bini A, Lazzari C & Palareti A (1995). Mortality among drug users in the AIDS era. *International Journal of Epidemiology*, **24**, 1204–10

Gold MS (1993). Opiate addiction and the locus coeruleus. *Psychiatric Clinics of North America*, **16**, 61–73

Gold MS, Pottash AC, Sweeney DR, Extein I & Annitto WJ (1981). Opiate detoxification with lofexidine. *Drug and Alcohol Dependence*, **8**, 307–15

Gonzalez JP & Brogden RN (1988). Naltrexone: a review of its pharmacodynamic and pharmacokinetic properties and therapeutic efficacy in the management of opioid dependence. *Drugs*, **35**, 192–213

Gorelick DA (1997). Enhancing cocaine metabolism with butyrylcholinesterase as a treatment strategy. *Drug and Alcohol Dependence*, **48**, 159–165

Gossop M (1988). Clonidine and the treatment of the opiate withdrawal syndrome. *Drug and Alcohol Dependence*, **21**, 253–9

Gossop M & Grant M (1991). A six country survey of the content and structure of heroin treatment programmes using methadone. *British Journal of Addiction*, **86**, 1151–60

Gossop M & Strang J (1991). A comparison of the withdrawal responses of heroin and methadone addicts during detoxification. *British Journal of Psychiatry*, **158**, 697–9

Gossop M, Johns A & Green L (1986). Opiate withdrawal: inpatient versus outpatient programmes and preferred versus random assignment to treatment. *British Medical Journal*, **293**, 103–4

Gossop M, Bradley M & Philips G (1987). An investigation of withdrawal symptoms shown by opiate addicts during and subsequent to a 21–day inpatient methadone detoxification. *Addictive Behaviours*, **12**, 1–6

Gossop M, Griffiths P, Bradley M & Strang J (1989). Opiate withdrawal symptoms in response to 10–day and 21–day methadone withdrawal programmes. *British Journal of Psychiatry*, **154**, 360–3

Gossop M, Battersby M & Strang J (1991). Self-detoxification by opiate addicts: a preliminary investigation. *British Journal of Psychiatry*, **159**, 208–12

Gossop M, Marsden J, Stewart D, Lehmann P, Edwards C, Wilson A & Segar G (1998). Substance use, health and social problems of service users at 54 drug treatment agencies: intake data from the National Treatment Outcome Research Study. *British Journal of Psychiatry*, **173**, 166–71

Grabowski J, Rhodes H, Elk, R, Schmitz J, Davis C, Creson D & Kirby K (1995). Fluoxetine is ineffective for treatment of cocaine dependence or concurrent opiate and cocaine dependence: two placebo-controlled, double-blind trials. *Journal of Clinical Psychopharmacology*, **15**, 163–74

Green L & Gossop M (1988). Effects of information on the opiate withdrawal syndrome. *British Journal of Addiction*, **83**, 305–9

Greenwood J (1992). Unpopular patients. *Druglink*, July/August, 8–10

Greenwood J (1996). Six years of sharing the care of Edinburgh drug users. *Psychiatric Bulletin*, **20**, 8–11

Griffin ML, Weiss RD, Mirin SM, Wilson H & Bouchard-Voelk B (1987). The use of the Diagnostic Interview Schedule in drug-dependent patients. *American Journal of Drug and*

*Alcohol Abuse*, **13**, 281–91

Griffiths RR & Weerts EM (1997). Benzodiazepine self-administration in humans and laboratory animals – implications for problems of long-term use and abuse. *Psychopharmacology*, **134**, 1–37

Gronbladh L, Ohlund LS & Gunne LM (1990). Mortality in heroin addiction: impact of methadone treatment. *Acta Psychiatrica Scandinavica*, **82**, 223–7

Gruer L, Wilson P, Scott R, Elliott L, Macleod J, Harden K, Forrester E, Hinshelwood S, McNulty H & Silk P (1997). General practitioner centred scheme for treatment of opiate dependent drug injectors in Glasgow. *British Medical Journal*, **314**, 1730–5

Grund JPC, Blanken P, Adriaans NFP, Kaplan CD, Barendregt C & Meenwsen M (1992). Reaching the unreached: an outreach model for 'on the spot' AIDS prevention among active, out-of-treatment drug addicts. In: O'Hare P, Newcombe R, Matthews A, Buning E & Drucker E. (eds.) *The Reduction of Drug-Related Harm* London: Routledge, pp. 172–80

Gunne LM & Gronbladh L (1981). The Swedish methadone maintenance program: a controlled study. *Drug and Alcohol Dependence*, **7**, 249–56

Hagopian GS, Wolfe HM, Sokol RJ, Ager JW, Wardell JN & Cepeda EE (1996). Neonatal outcome following methadone exposure in utero. *The Journal of Maternal–Fetal Medicine*, **5**, 348–54

Hajek P (1996). Current issues in behavioural and pharmacological approaches to smoking cessation. *Addictive Behaviors*, **21**, 699–707

Halikas JA, Kuhn KL, Crea FS, Carlson GA & Crosby R (1992). Treatment of crack cocaine use with carbamazepine. *American Journal of Drug and Alcohol Abuse*, **18**, 45–56

Hall W & Farrell (1997). Comorbidity of mental disorders with substance misuse. *British Journal of Psychiatry*, **171**, 4–5

Hall W & Solowij N (1997). Long-term cannabis use and mental health. *British Journal of Psychiatry*, **171**, 107–8

Hall W, Solowij N & Lemon J (1996). Australian National Drug Strategy Monograph No 25. 'The Health and Psychological Consequences of Cannabis Use' (extract). *Addiction*, **91**, 759–62

Hall W, Ward J & Mattick RP (1998). The effectiveness of methadone maintenance treatment. 1: Heroin use and crime. In: Ward J, Mattick RP & Hall W (eds.) *Methadone Maintenance Treatment and Other Opioid Replacement Therapies*, London: Harwood, pp. 17–58

Hammersley R, Cassidy MR & Oliver J (1995). Drugs associated with drug-related deaths in Edinburgh and Glasgow, November 1990 to October 1992. *Addiction*, **90**, 959–65

Hando J, Flaherty B & Rutter S (1997). An Australian profile on the use of cocaine. *Addiction*, **92**, 173–82

Harrison M, Busto U, Naranjo CA, Kaplan HL & Sellers EM (1984). Diazepam tapering in detoxification for high dose benzodiazepine abuse. *Clinical Pharmacology and Therapeutics*, **36**, 527–33

Hartel DM, Schoenbaum EE, Selwyn PA, Kline J, Davenny K, Klein RS & Friedland GH (1995). Heroin use during methadone maintenance treatment: the importance of methadone dose and cocaine use. *American Journal of Public Health*, **85**, 83–8

Hartnoll RL, Mitcheson MC, Battersby A, Brown G, Ellis M, Fleming P & Hedley N (1980). Evaluation of heroin maintenance in controlled trial. *Archives of General Psychiatry*, **37**, 877–84

Haugland G, Siegel C, Alexander MJ & Galanter M (1991). A survey of hospitals in New York State treating psychiatric patients with chemical abuse disorders. *Hospital and Community Psychiatry*, **42**, 1215–20

Haverkos HW & Stein MD (1995). Identifying substance abuse in primary care. *American Family Physician*, **52**, 2029–35

Hawkes D, Mitcheson M, Osborne A & Edwards G (1969). Abuse of methylamphetamine. *British Medical Journal*, **2**, 715–21

Haynes B & Haines A (1998). Barriers and bridges to evidence based clinical practice. *British Medical Journal*, **317**, 273–6

Haywood TW, Kravitz HM, Grossman LS, Cavanaugh JL, Davis JM & Lewis DA (1995). Predicting the 'revolving door' phenomenon among patients with schizophrenic, schizoaffective and affective disorders. *American Journal of Psychiatry*, **152**, 856–61

Hellawell K (1995). The role of law enforcement in minimising the harm resulting from illicit drugs. *Drug and Alcohol Review*, **14**, 317–22

Henningfield JE (1995). Nicotine medications for smoking cessation. *New England Journal of Medicine*, **333**, 1196–203

Henry JA, Jeffreys KJ & Dawling S (1992). Toxicity and deaths from 3,4–methylene-dioxymethamphetamine ('ecstasy'). *The Lancet*, **340**, 384–7

Higgins ST, Budney AJ, Bickel WK, Foerg FE, Donham R & Badger GJ (1994a). Incentives improve outcome in outpatient behavioural treatment of cocaine dependence. *Archives of General Psychiatry*, **51**, 568–76

Higgins ST, Budney AJ, Bickel WK & Badger MS (1994b). Participation of significant others in outpatient behavioural treatment predicts greater cocaine abstinence. *American Journal of Drug and Alcohol Abuse*, **20**, 47–56

Hoffman JA, Moolchan ET & Rodriguez SM (1996). Tobacco addiction. *Current Opinion in Psychiatry*, **9**, 221–4

Hubbard RL, Rachal JV, Craddock SG & Cavanagh ER (1984). Treatment Outcome Prospective Study (TOPS): client characteristics and behaviours before, during, and after treatment. In: Timms FM & Ludford JP (eds.) *Drug Abuse Treatment Evaluation: Strategies, Progress and Prospects*, NIDA Research Monograph No. 51

Hubbard RL, Marsden ME, Rachal JV, Harwood HJ, Cavanagh ER & Ginzburg HM (1989). *Drug Abuse Treatment: A National Study of Effectiveness*. University of North Carolina Press

Hughes JR (1996). The future of smoking cessation therapy in the United States. *Addiction*, **91**, 1797–802

Hulse GK, Milne G, English DR & Holman CDJ (1997). Assessing the relationship between maternal cocaine use and abruptio placentae. *Addiction*, **92**, 1547–51

Iguchi MY, Handelsman L, Bickel WK & Griffiths RR (1993). Benzodiazepine and sedative use/abuse by methadone maintenance clients.. *Drug and Alcohol Dependence*, **32**, 257–66

Jarvis MAE & Schnoll SH (1994). Methadone treatment during pregnancy. *Journal of Psychoactive Drugs*, **26**, 155–61

Jaudes PK, Ekwo E & van Voorhis J (1995). Association of drug abuse and child abuse. *Child Abuse and Neglect*, **19**, 1065–75

Jerrell JM & Ridgeley MS (1995). Comparative effectiveness of three approaches to serving people with severe mental illness and substance abuse disorders. *Journal of Nervous and Mental Disease*, **183**, 566–76

Joe GW, Simpson DD & Hubbard RL (1991). Treatment predictors of tenure in methadone maintenance. *Journal of Substance Abuse*, **3**, 73–84

Johnson RE, Eissenberg T, Stitzer ML, Strain EC, Liebson IA & Bigelow GE (1995). A placebo controlled clinical trial of buprenorphine as a treatment for opioid dependence. *Drug and Alcohol Dependence*, **40**, 17–25

Johnson S (1997). Dual diagnosis of severe mental illness and substance misuse: a case for specialist services? *British Journal of Psychiatry*, **171**, 205–8

Joseph AM, Nichol KL, Willenbring ML, Korn JE & Lysaght LS (1990). Beneficial effects of treatment of nicotine dependence during an inpatient substance abuse treatment program. *Journal of the American Medical Association*, **263**, 3043–6

Kain ZN, Kain TS & Scarpelli EM (1992). Cocaine exposure in utero: perinatal development and neonatal manifestations – review. *Clinical Toxicology*, **30**, 607–36

Kalant H, Ghodse H, Chowdhury AN, Negrete JC & Hawks D (1996). Comments on Hall et al.'s Australian National Drug Strategy Monograph No. 25 'The Health and Psychological Consequences of Cannabis Use'. *Addiction*, **91**, 762–73

Kaltenbach K & Finnegan LP (1987). Perinatal and developmental outcome of infants exposed to methadone in-utero. *Neurotoxicology and Teratology*, **9**, 311–13

Kandel DB & Davies M (1992). Progression to regular marijuana involvement: phenomenology and risk factors for near daily use. In: Glanz M & Pickens R, *Vulnerability to Drug Abuse*, Washington: American Psychological Association, pp. 211–53

Kavoussi RJ, Liu J & Coccaro EF (1994). An open trial of sertraline in personality disordered patients with impulsive aggression. *Journal of Clinical Psychiatry*, **55**, 137–41

Khalsa ME, Paredes A, Anglin MD, Potepan P & Potter C (1993). *Combinations of treatment modalities and therapeutic outcome for cocaine dependence*. NIDA Research Monograph, **135**, 237–59

Khan A, Mumford JP, Ash Rogers G & Beckford H (1997). Double-blind study of lofexidine and clonidine in the detoxification of opiate addicts in hospital. *Drug and Alcohol Dependence*, **44**, 57–61

King L (1997). Structured GP liaison for substance misuse. *Nursing Times*, **93**, 30–1

Klee H (1992). A new target for behavioural research – amphetamine use. *British Journal of Addiction*, **87**, 439–46

Klee H, Faugier J, Hayes C, Boulton T & Morris J (1990). Aids-related risk behaviour, polydrug use and temazepam. *British Journal of Addiction*, **85**, 1125–32

Klingemann HKH (1996). Drug treatment in Switzerland: harm reduction, decentralisation and community response. *Addiction*, **91**, 723–36

Kolar AF, Brown BS, Haertzen CA & Michaelson BS (1994). Children of substance abusers: the life experiences of children of opiate addicts in methadone maintenance. *American Journal of Drug and Alcohol Abuse*, **20**, 159–71

Korkia P (1997). Anabolic–androgenic steroids and their uses in sport and recreation. *Journal of Substance Misuse*, **2**, 131–5

Kosten TA, Gawin FH, Kosten TR & Rounsaville BJ (1993). Gender differences in cocaine use and treatment response. *Journal of Substance Abuse Treatment*, **10**, 63–6

Krausz M, Verthein U, Degkwitz P, Haasen C & Raschke P (1998). Maintenance treatment of opiate addicts in Germany with medications containing codeine – results of a follow-up study. *Addiction*, **93**, 1161–7

Kreek MJ (1978). Medical complications in methadone patients. *Annals of the New York Academy of Sciences*, **311**, 110–34

Kreek MJ (1992). Rationale for maintenance pharmacotherapy of opiate dependence. In:

O'Brien CP & Jaffe JH (eds.) *Addictive States*. New York: Raven Press

Lader M (1993). Historical development of the concept of tranquillizer dependence. In: Hallstrom C (ed.) *Benzodiazepine Dependence*. Oxford: Oxford Medical Publications, pp. 46–57

Lader M (1997). Zopiclone: is there any dependence and abuse potential? *Journal of Neurology*, **244**, 518–22

Lader M & Morton S (1991). Benzodiazepine problems. *British Journal of Addiction*, **86**, 823–8

Landabaso MA, Iraurgi I, Jimenez-Lerma JM, Sanz J, Fernandez de Corres B, Araluce K, Calle R & Gutierrez-Fraile M (1998). A randomized trial of adding fluoxetine to a naltrexone treatment programme for heroin addicts. *Addiction*, **93**, 739–44

Lavelle T, Hammersley R, Forsyth A & Bain D (1991). The use of buprenorphine and temazepam by drug injectors. *Journal of Addictive Diseases*, **10**, 5–14

Law FD, Bailey JE, Allen DS, Melichar JK, Myles JS, Mitcheson MC, Lewis JW & Nutt DJ (1997). The feasibility of abrupt methadone–buprenorphine transfer in British opiate addicts in an outpatient setting. *Addiction Biology*, **2**, 191–200

Leaver EJ, Elford J, Morris JK & Cohen J (1992). Use of general practice by intravenous heroin users on a methadone programme. *British Journal of General Practice*, **42**, 465–8

Lehman AF, Myeers CP, Thompson JW & Corty E (1993a). Implications of mental and substance use disorders: a comparison of single and dual diagnosis patients. *Journal of Nervous and Mental Disease*, **181**, 365–70

Lehman AF, Herron JD, Schwartz RP et al. (1993b). Rehabilitation for adults with severe mental illness and substance abuse disorders: a clinical trial. *Journal of Nervous and Mental Disease*, **181**, 86–90

Levin FR & Lehman AF (1991). Meta-analysis of desipramine as an adjunct in the treatment of cocaine addiction. *Journal of Clinical Psychopharmacology*, **11**, 371–8

Lewis B, McCusker J, Hindin R, Frost R & Garfield F (1993). Four residential drug treatment programs: Project IMPACT. In: Inciardi J, Tims F & Fletcher B (eds.) *Innovative Strategies in the Treatment of Drug Abuse*. Westport, CTL: Greenwood Publishers, pp. 45–60

Liappas JA, Jenner FA, Vlissides DNH & Vicente B (1987). Thoughts on the Sheffield non-prescribing programme for narcotic users. *British Journal of Addictions*, **82**, 999–1006

Lin SK, Strang J, Su LW, Tsai CJ & Hu WH (1997). Double-blind randomised controlled trial of lofexidine versus clonidine in the treatment of heroin withdrawal. *Drug and Alcohol Dependence*, **48**, 127–33

Ling W, Charuvastra C, Kaim SC & Klett CJ (1976). Methadyl acetate and methadone as maintenance treatments for heroin addicts. *Archives of General Psychiatry*, **33**, 709–20

Ling W, Rawson RA & Compton MA (1994). Substitution pharmacotherapies for opioid addiction: from methadone to LAAM and buprenorphine. *Journal of Psychoactive Drugs*, **26**, 119–28

Ling W, Charuvastra C, Collins JF, Barki S, Brown LS, Kintaudi P et al. (1998). Buprenorphine maintenance treatment of opiate dependence: a multicenter, randomized clinical trial. *Addiction*, **93**, 475–86

Lipton DS, Brewington V & Smith M (1994). Acupuncture for crack cocaine detoxification: experimental evaluation of efficacy. *Journal of Substance Abuse Treatment*, **11**, 205–15

Loimer N, Lenz, Schmid R & Presslich O (1991a). Technique for greatly shortening the transition from methadone to naltrexone maintenance of patients addicted to opiates. *American Journal of Psychiatry*, **148**, 933–5

Loimer N, Schmid R, Grunberger J, Jaggch R, Linzmayer L & Presslich O (1991b). Psychophysiological reactions in methadone maintenance patients do not correlate with methadone plasma levels. *Psychopharmacology*, **103**, 538–40

Lowinson J, Berle B & Langrod J (1976). Detoxification of long-term methadone patients: problems and prospects. *International Journal of the Addictions*, **11**, 1009–18

Maas U, Kattner E, Weingart-Hesse B, Schafter A & Obladen M (1990). Infrequent neonatal opiate withdrawal following maternal methadone detoxification during pregnancy. *Journal of Perinatal Medicine*, **18**, 111–18

Mack G, Thomas D, Giles W & Buchanan N (1991). Methadone levels and neonatal withdrawal. *Journal of Paediatrics and Child Health*, **27**, 96–100

MacLeod J, Whittaker A & Robertson JR (1998). Changes in opiate treatment during attendance at a community drug service – findings from a clinical audit. *Drug and Alcohol Review*, **17**, 19–25

Magura S, Rosenblum A, Lovejoy M, Handelsman L, Foote J & Stimmel B (1994). Neurobehavioural treatment for cocaine-using methadone patients: a preliminary report. *Journal of Addictive Diseases*, **13**, 143–60

Malpas RJ, Darlow BA, Lennox R & Horwood LJ (1995). Maternal methadone dosage and neonatal withdrawal. *Australian and New Zealand Journal of Obstetrics and Gynaecology*, **35**, 175–7

Mant A & Walsh RA (1997). Reducing benzodiazepine use. *Drug and Alcohol Review*, **16**, 77–84

Markowitz PJ, Calabrese JR, Schulz SC & Meltzer HY (1991). Fluoxetine in the treatment of borderline and schizotypal personality disorder. *American Journal of Psychiatry*, **148**, 1064–7

Marks J (1994). Deaths from methadone and heroin. *Lancet*, **343**, 976

Marks J (1996). Accidy, addiction and the prohibition. *Addiction Research*, **4**, i–v (editorial)

Marks J, Palombella A & Newcombe R (1991). The smoking option. *Druglink*, May/June, 10–11

Marlatt GA & Gordon JR (eds.) (1985). *Relapse Prevention: Maintenance Strategies in the Treatment of Addictive Behaviours*. New York: Guilford Press

Marsch LA (1998). The efficacy of methadone maintenance interventions in reducing illicit opiate use, HIV risk behaviour and criminality: a meta-analysis. *Addiction*, **93**, 515–32

Mattick RP & Hall W (1996). Are detoxification programmes effective? *Lancet*, **347**, 97–100

Maxwell DL, Polkey MI & Henry JA (1993). Hyponatraemia and catatonic stupor after taking 'ecstasy'. *British Medical Journal*, **307**, 1399

McCann UD & Ricaurte GA (1992). MDMA ('Ecstasy') and panic disorder: induction by a single dose. *Biological Psychiatry*, **32**, 950–53

McCann UD, Ridenour A, Shaham Y & Ricaurte GA (1994). Serotonin neurotoxicity after ( ±)3, 4–Methylenedioxymethamphetamine (MDMA;'Ecstasy'): a controlled study in humans. *Neuropsychopharmacology*, **10**, 129–38

McDuff DR, Schwartz RP, Tommasello A, Tiegel S, Conovan T & Johnson JL (1993). Outpatient benzodiazepine detoxification procedure for methadone patients. *Journal of Substance Abuse Treatment*, **10**, 297–302

McGlothin WH & Anglin MD (1981). Long-term follow-up of clients of high- and low-dose methadone programs. *Archives of General Psychiatry*, **38**, 1055–63

McLachlan C, Crofts N, Wodak A & Crowe S (1993). The effects of methadone on immune function among injecting drug users: a review. *Addiction*, **88**, 257–63

McLean PC & Casey P (1982). Drugs of dependence. In: Tyrer PJ (ed.) *Drugs in Psychiatric Practice*. London: Butterworths, pp. 321–51

McLellan AT, Childress AR, Ehrman R, O'Brien CP & Pashko S (1986). Extinguishing conditioned responses during opiate dependence treatment: turning laboratory findings into clinical procedures. *Journal of Substance Abuse Treatment*, **3**, 33–40

McLellan AT, Arndt IO, Metzger DS, Woody GE & O'Brien CP (1993). The effects of psychosocial services in substance abuse treatment. *Journal of the American Medical Association*, **269**, 1953–9

McMahon RC, Lelley A & Kouzekanani K (1993). Personality and coping styles in the prediction of dropout from treatment for cocaine abuse. *Journal of Personality Assessment*, **61**, 147–55

McPhillips MA, Strang J & Barnes TRE (1998). Hair analysis. New laboratory ability to test for substance use. *British Journal of Psychiatry*, **173**, 287–90

Mello NK & Mendelson JH (1985). Behavioural pharmacology of buprenorphine. *Drug and Alcohol Dependence*, **14**, 283–303

Mendoza R & Miller B (1992). Neuropsychiatric disorders associated with cocaine use. *Hospital and Community Psychiatry*, **43**, 677–80

Menezes PR, Johnson S, Thornicroft G, Marshall J, Prosser D, Bebbington P & Kuipers E (1996). Drug and alcohol problems among individuals with severe mental illness in South London. *British Journal of Psychiatry*, **168**, 612–19

Merrill J & Marshall R (1997). Opioid detoxification using naloxone. *Drug and Alcohol Review*, **16**, 3–6

Merrill J, Garvey T & Rosson C (1996). Methadone concentrations taken as indicating deaths due to overdose need to be reviewed. *British Medical Journal*, **313**, 1481

Metrebian N, Shanahan W & Stimson GV (1996). Heroin prescribing in the United Kingdom: an overview. *European Addiction Research*, **2**, 194–200

Metzer DS, Woody GE, McLellan AT, O'Brien CP, Druley P, Navaline H, De Phillipis D, Stolley P & Abrutyn E (1993). Human immunodeficiency virus seroconversion among intravenous drug users in- and out-of-treatment: an eighteen month prospective follow-up. *Journal of the Acquired Immune Deficiency Syndrome*, **6**, 1049–56

Milby JB, Gurwitch RH, Wiebe DJ, Ling W, McLellan AT & Woody GE (1986). Prevalence and diagnostic reliability of methadone maintenance detoxification fear. *American Journal of Psychiatry*, **143**, 739–43

Miller P (1997). Family structure, personality, drinking, smoking and illicit drug use: a study of UK teenagers. *Drugs and Alcohol Dependence*, **45**, 121–9

Milroy CM, Clark JC & Forrest ARW (1996). Pathology of deaths associated with 'ecstasy' and 'eve' misuse. *Journal of Clinical Pathology*, **49**, 149–53

Monti PM, Rohsenow DJ, Michalec E, Martin RA & Abrams DB (1997). Brief coping skills treatment for cocaine abuse: substance use outcomes at three months. *Addiction*, **92**, 1717–28

Montoya ID, Levin FR, Fudala PJ et al. (1995). Double-blind comparison of carbamazepine and placebo for treatment of cocaine dependence. *Drug and Alcohol Dependence*, **38**, 213

Morrison CL & Ruben SM (1995). The development of health care services for drug misusers and prostitutes. *Postgraduate Medical Journal*, **71**, 593–7

Mos J & Oliver B (1987). Pro-aggressive actions of benzodiazepines. In: Oliver B, Mos J & Brain PF (eds.) *Ethopharmacology of Agonistic Behaviour in Animals and Humans*. Dordrecht: Martinus Nijhoff, pp. 187–206

Mueser KT, Drake RE, Alterman AI & Ackerson TH (1997). Antisocial personality disorder, conduct disorder, and substance abuse in schizophrenia. *Journal of Abnormal Psychology*, **106**, 473–7

Musselman DL & Kell MJ (1995). Prevalence and improvement in psychopathology in opioid dependent patients participating in methadone maintenance. *Journal of Addictive Diseases*, **14**, 67–82

Myles J (1997). Treatment for amphetamine use in the United Kingdom . In: Klee H (ed.) *Amphetamine Misuse, International Perspectives on Current Trends*. The Netherlands: Harwood Academic Publishers, pp. 69–79

Nathan KI, Bresnick WH & Batki SL (1998). Cocaine abuse and dependence. Approaches to management. *CNS Drugs*, **10**, 43–59

Negus SS & Woods JH (1995). Reinforcing effects, discriminative stimulus effects, and physical dependence liability of buprenorphine. In: Cowan A & Lewis JW (eds.) *Buprenorphine: Combatting Drug Abuse with a Unique Opioid*. New York: Wiley-Liss, pp. 71–101

Newman RG & Whitehill WB (1979). Double-blind comparison of methadone and placebo maintenance treatments of narcotic addicts in Hong Kong. *Lancet*, **2**, 485–8

Ng B & Alvear M (1993). Dextropropoxyphene Addiction – a drug of primary abuse. *American Journal of Drug and Alcohol Abuse*, **19**, 153–8

Noonan WC & Moyers TB (1997). Motivational interviewing. *Journal of Substance Misuse*, **2**, 8–16

Norden MJ (1989). Fluoxetine in borderline personality disorder: progress in neuropharmacology. *Biological Psychiatry*, **13**, 343–53

Novick DM & Joseph H (1991). Medical maintenance: the treatment of chronic opiate dependence in general medical practice. *Journal of Substance Abuse Treatment*, **8**, 233–9

Novick DM, Richman BL, Friendman JM, Friendman JE, Fried C, Wilson JP et al. (1993). The medical status of methadone maintenance patients in treatment for 11–18 years. *Drug and Alcohol Dependence*, **33**, 235–45

O'Brien CP (1996). Recent developments in the pharmacotherapy of substance abuse. *Journal of Consulting and Clinical Psychology*, **64**, 677–86

O'Brien CP, Childress AP, McLellan T et al. (1990). Integrating systemic cue exposure with standard treatment in recovering drug dependent patients. *Addictive Behaviours*, **15**, 355–65

Oppenheimer E, Robutt C, Taylor C & Andrew T (1994). Death and survival in a cohort of heroin addicts from London clinics: a 22-year follow-up study. *Addiction*, **89**, 1299–308

Paris J (1996a). Social factors – mechanisms. In: *Social Factors in the Personality Disorders: A biopsychosocial approach to aetiology and treatment*. Cambridge: Cambridge University Press, pp. 73–94

Paris J (1996b). Psychological factors. In: *Social Factors in the Personality Disorders: A biopsychosocial approach to aetiology and treatment*. Cambridge: Cambridge University Press, pp. 40–63

Patton LH (1995). Adolescent substance abuse. *Pediatric Clinics of North America*, **42**,

283–93

Payne-James JJ, Dean PJ & Keys DW (1994). Drug misusers in police custody: a prospective survey. *Journal of the Royal Society of Medicine*, **87**, 13–14

Pearson G (1996). Drugs and deprivation. *Journal of the Royal Society of Health*, April, 113–16

Perkins KA (1996). Sex differences in nicotine versus nonnicotine reinforcement as determinants of tobacco smoking. *Experimental and Clinical Psychopharmacology*, **4**, 166–77

Peroutka SJ, Newman H & Harris H (1988). Subjective effects of 3, 4–methylenedioxymethamphetamine in recreational users. *Neuropsychopharmacology*, **1**, 273–7

Petursson H & Lader MH (1981). Withdrawal from long-term benzodiazepine treatment. *British Medical Journal*, **238**, 643–5

Philips G, Gossop M & Bradley M (1986). The influence of psychological factors on the opiate withdrawal syndrome. *British Journal of Psychiatry*, **149**, 135–8

Plomp HN, van der Hek H & Ader HJ (1996). The Amsterdam Methadone Dispensing Circuit: genesis and effectiveness of a public health model for local drug policy. *Addiction*, **91**, 711–21

Pollack M & Rosenbaum J (1991). Fluoxetine treatment of cocaine abuse in heroin addicts. *Journal of Clinical Psychiatry*, **52**, 31–3

Pollack M, Brotman A & Rosenbaum J (1989). Cocaine abuse treatment. *Comprehensive Psychiatry*, **30**, 31–44

Polson RG, Fleming PM & O'Shea JK (1993). Fluoxetine in the treatment of amphetamine dependence. *Human Psychopharmacology*, **8**, 55–8

Poole R & Brabbins C (1996). Drug induced psychosis. *British Journal of Psychiatry*, **168**, 135–8

Poulton G & Andrews G (1992). Personality as a cause of adverse life events. *Acta Psychiatrica Scandinavica*, **85**, 35–8

Preston A (1996a). *The Methadone Briefing*, pp. 42–50. London: Island Press/Institute for Study of Drug Dependence

Preston A (1996b). *The Methadone Briefing*, pp. 108–11. London: Island Press/Institute for Study of Drug Dependence

Preston A (1996c). *The Methadone Briefing*, p. 16. London: Island Press/Institute for Study of Drug Dependence

Preston KL, Griffiths RR, Stitzer ML, Bigelow GE & Liebson IA (1984). Diazepam and methadone interactions in methadone maintenance. *Clinical Pharmacology and Therapeutics*, **36**, 534–41

Raistrick D (1994). Report of Advisory Council on the Misuse of Drugs: AIDS and Drug Misuse Update. *Addiction*, **89**, 1211–13

Raistrick D (1997). Substitute prescribing – social policy or individual treatment? (and why we must make the decision). *Druglink*, March/April, 16–17

Ralston GE & Kidd BA (1996). General practitioners and drug users: their current practice and expectations of specialist service. *Health Bulletin*, **54**, 16–21

Rawson RA, Obert J, McCann MJ, Castro FG & Ling W (1991). Cocaine abuse treatment: a review of current strategies. *Journal of Substance Abuse*, **3**, 457–91

Rawson RA, McCann MJ, Hasson AJ & Ling W (1994). Cocaine abuse among methadone maintenance patients: are there effective treatment strategies? *Journal of Psychoactive Drugs*, **26**, 129–36

Rawson RA, Hasson AJ, Huber AM, McCann MJ & Ling W (1998). A 3–year progress report on the implementation of LAAM in the United States. *Addiction*, **93**, 533–40

Regier DA, Farmer ME, Rae DS, Locke BZ, Keith SJ, Judd LL & Goodwin FK (1990). Comorbidity of mental disorders with alcohol and other drug abuse. *Journal of the American Medical Association*, **264**, 2511–18

Reich JH & Vasile RG (1993). Effect of personality disorders on the treatment outcome of Axis I conditions: an update. *Journal of Nervous and Mental Disease*, **181**, 475–83

Reisinger M (1997). Use of buprenorphine during pregnancy. *Research and Clinical Forums*, **19 (2)**, 43–5

Reynaud M, Petit G, Potard D & Courty P (1998). Six deaths linked to concomitant use of buprenorphine and benzodiazepines. *Addiction*, **93**, 1385–92

Richardson MP & Sharland M (1998). Late diagnosis of paediatric HIV infection in south west London. *British Medical Journal*, **316**, 271–2

Ries RK, Roy-Byrne PP, Ward NG, Neppe V & Cullison S (1989). Carbamazepine treatment for benzodiazepine withdrawal. *American Journal of Psychiatry*, **146**, 536–7

Ripple CH & Luthar SS (1996). Familial factors in illicit drug abuse: an interdisciplinary perspective. *American Journal of Drug and Alcohol Abuse*, **22**, 147–72

Risser D & Schneider B (1994). Drug-related deaths between 1985 and 1992 examined at the Institute of Forensic Medicine in Vienna, Austria. *Addiction*, **89**, 851–7

Robertson JR (1989). Treatment of drug misuse in the general practice setting. *British Journal of Addiction*, **84**, 377–80

Robson P & Bruce M (1997). A comparison of 'visible' and 'invisible' users of amphetamine, cocaine and heroin: two distinct populations? *Addiction*, **92**, 1729–36

Ronald PJM, Witcomb JC, Robertson JR, Roberts JJK, Shishodia PC & Whittaker A (1992). Problems of drug abuse, HIV and AIDS: the burden of care in one general practice. *British Journal of General Practice*, **42**, 232–5

Rosen M & Kosten TR (1995). Detoxification and induction onto naltrexone. In: Cowan A & Lewis JW (eds.) *Buprenorphine: Combatting Drug Abuse with a Unique Opioid*. New York: Wiley-Liss, pp. 289–305

Rosenbaum M (1995). The demedicalization of methadone maintenance. *Journal of Psychoactive Drugs*, **27**, 145–9

Rosenbaum M & Murphy S (1984). Always a junkie?: The arduous task of getting off methadone maintenance. *Journal of Drug Issues*, **14**, 527–52

Rosenbaum M, Irwin J & Murphy S (1988). De facto destabilisation as policy: the impact of short-term methadone maintenance. *Contemporary Drug Problems*, **15**, 491–517

Ross HE, Glaser FB & Germanson T (1988). The prevalence of psychiatric disorders in patients with alcohol and other drug problems. *Archives of General Psychiatry*, **45**, 1023–31

Ross J, Darke S & Hall W (1997). Transitions between routes of benzodiazepine administration among heroin users in Sydney. *Addiction*, **92**, 697–705

Rounsaville BJ, Weissman MM, Kleber H & Wilber C (1982). Heterogeneity of psychiatric diagnosis in treated opiate addicts. *Archives of General Psychiatry*, **39**, 161–6

Rounsaville BJ, Glazer W, Wilber CH, Weissman MM & Kleber HD (1983). Short-term interpersonal psychotherapy in methadone-maintained opiate addicts. *Archives of General Psychiatry*, **40**, 629–36

Ruben SM & Morrison CL (1992). Temazepam misuse in a group of injecting drug users. *British Journal of Addiction*, **87**, 1387–92

Ruben SM, McLean PC & Melville J (1989). Cyclizine abuse among a group of opiate dependents receiving methadone. *British Journal of Addiction*, **84**, 929–34

Rumball D & Williams J (1997). Rapid opiate detoxification. *British Medical Journal*, **315**, 682

Salazar C (1997). Relapse prevention and nursing interventions. In: Rassool GH & Gafoor M (eds.) *Addiction Nursing. Perspectives on Professional and Clinical Practice*. Gloucester: Stanley Thornes, pp. 67–79

San L, Cami J, Peri JM, Mata R & Porta M (1990). Efficacy of clonidine, guanfacine and methadone in the rapid detoxification of heroin addicts: a controlled clinical trial. *British Journal of Addiction*, **85**, 141–7

San L, Pomarol G, Peri JM, Olle JM & Cami J (1991). Follow-up after a six-month maintenance period of naltrexone versus placebo in heroin addicts. *British Journal of Addiction*, **86**, 983–90

San L, Fernandez T, Cami J & Gossop M (1994). Efficacy of methadone versus methadone and guanfacine in the detoxification of heroin-addicted patients. *Journal of Substance Abuse Treatment*, **11**, 463–9

Sass H, Soyka M, Mann K & Zieglgansberger W (1996). Relapse prevention by acamprosate: Results from a placebo-controlled study on alcohol dependence. *Archives of General Psychiatry*, **53**, 673–80

Saunders B, Wilkinson C & Phillips M (1995). The impact of a brief motivational intervention with opiate users attending a methadone programme. *Addiction*, **90**, 415–24

Saxon AJ, McGuffin R & Walker RD (1997). An open trial of transdermal nicotine replacement therapy for smoking cessation among alcohol- and drug-dependent inpatients. *Journal of Substance Abuse Treatment*, **14**, 333–7

Scally G & Donaldson LJ (1998). The NHS's 50th anniversary: clinical governance and the drive for quality improvement in the new NHS in England. *British Medical Journal*, **317**, 61–5

Scott H, Johnson S, Menezes P, Thornicroft G, Marshall J, Bindman J et al. (1998). Substance misuse and risk of aggression and offending among the severely mentally ill. *British Journal of Psychiatry*, **172**, 345–50

Scott R (1990). The prevention of convulsions during benzodiazepine withdrawals. *British Journal of General Practice*, **40**, 261

Scott R (1996). Shared care. Pharmacists work. *Druglink*, Jan/Feb, 13–14

Seivewright N (1987). Relationships between life events and personality in psychiatric disorder. *Stress Medicine*, **3**, 163–8

Seivewright N (1998). Theory and practice in managing benzodiazepine dependence and abuse. *Journal of Substance Misuse*, **3**, 170–7

Seivewright N & Dougal W (1993). Withdrawal symptoms from high dose benzodiazepines in poly drug users. *Drug and Alcohol Dependence*, **32**, 15–23

Seivewright N & Greenwood J (1996). What is important in drug misuse treatment? *Lancet*, **347**, 373–6

Seivewright N & McMahon C (1996). Misuse of amphetamines and related drugs. *Advances in Psychiatric Treatment*, **2**, 211–18

Seivewright N & Daly C (1997). Personality disorder and drug use: a review. *Drug and Alcohol Review*, **16**, 235–50

Seivewright N, Donmall M & Daly C (1993). Benzodiazepines in the illicit drug scene – the

UK picture and some treatment dilemmas. *International Journal of Drug Policy*, **4**, 42–8

Sell L, Farrell M & Robson P (1997). Prescription of diamorphine, dipipanone and cocaine in England and Wales. *Drug and Alcohol Review*, **16**, 221–6

Sellers EM, Higgins GA, Tomkins DR, Romach MK & Toneatto T (1991). Opportunities for treatment of psychoactive substance use disorders with serotonergic medications. *Journal of Clinical Psychiatry*, **52**:12 (Supp), 49–54

Senay EC, Barthwell AG, Marks R, Bokos P, Gillman D & White R (1993). Medical maintenance: a pilot study. *Journal of Addictive Diseases*, **12**, 59–75

Seow SW, Swensen G, Willis D, Hartfield M & Chapman C (1980). Extraneous drug use in methadone-supported patients. *Medical Journal of Australia*, **1**, 269–71

Serfaty MA, Lawrie A, Smith B, Brind AM, Watson JP, Gilvarry E & Bassendine MF (1997). Risk factors and medical follow-up of drug users tested for hepatitis C – can the risk of transmission be reduced? *Drug and Alcohol Review*, **16**, 339–47

Shaner A, Eckman TA, Roberts LJ, Wilkins JN, Tucker D, Tsuang JW et al. (1995). Disability income, cocaine use and repeated hospitalisation among schizophrenic cocaine abusers: a government-sponsored revolving door? *New England Journal of Medicine*, **333**, 777–83

Shepherd RT (1989). Mechanism of sudden death associated with volatile substance abuse. *Human Toxicology*, **8**, 287–91

Sherman JP (1990). Dexamphetamine for 'speed' addiction. *Medical Journal of Australia*, **153**, 306

Shufman EN, Porat S, Witztum E, Gandacu D, Bar-Hamburger R & Ginath Y (1994). The efficacy of naltrexone in preventing re-abuse of heroin after detoxification. *Society of Biological Psychiatry*, **35**, 935–45

Silverman K, Higgins ST, Brooner RK, Montoya ID, Cone EJ, Schuster CR & Preston KL (1996). Sustained cocaine abstinence in methadone maintenance patients through voucher-based reinforcement therapy. *Archives of General Psychiatry*, **53**, 409–15

Solowij N (1993). Ecstasy (3,4–methylenedioxymethamphetamine). *Current Opinion in Psychiatry*, **6**, 411–15

Spring WD, Willenbring ML & Maddux TL (1992). Sexual dysfunction and psychological distress in methadone maintenance. *International Journal of the Addictions*, **27**, 1325–34

Stark K, Muller K, Bienzle U & Guggenmoos-Holzmann I (1996). Methadone maintenance treatment and HIV risk-taking behaviour among injecting drug users in Berlin. *Journal of Epidemiology and Community Health*, **50**, 534–7

Steele C (1995). Helping patients to stop smoking. *Practitioner*, **239**, 154–6

Steels MD, Hamilton M & McLean PC (1992). The consequences of a change in formulation of methadone prescribed in a drug clinic. *British Journal of Addiction*, **87**, 1549–54

Stephens RS, Roffman RA & Simpson EE (1993). Adult marijuana users seeking treatment. *Journal of Consulting and Clinical Psychology*, **61**, 110–14

Stimson GV (1996). Has the United Kingdom averted an epidemic of HIV-I infection among drug injectors? *Addiction*, **91**, 1085–8

Stitzer ML, Griffiths RR, McLellan AT, Graboswki J & Hawthorne JW (1981). Diazepam use among methadone patients: patterns and dosages. *Drug and Alcohol Dependence*, **8**, 189–99

Stitzer ML, Bigelow GE, Liebson IA & Hawthorne JW (1982). Contingent reinforcement for benzodiazepine-free urines: evaluation of a drug abuse treatment intervention.

*Journal of Applied Behavioural Analysis*, **15**, 493–503

Stolerman IP & Jarvis MJ (1995). The scientific case that nicotine is addictive. *Psychopharmacology*, **117**, 2–10

Strain EC, Stitzer ML, Liebson IA & Bigelow GE (1994a). Comparison of buprenorphine and methadone in the treatment of opioid dependence. *American Journal of Psychiatry*, **151**, 1025–30

Strain EC, Stitzer ML, Liebson IA & Bigelow GE (1994b). Buprenorphine versus methadone in the treatment of opioid-dependent cocaine users. *Psychopharmacology*, **116**, 401–6

Strang J & Farrell M (1992). Harm minimization for drug insurers. When second best may be best first. *British Medical Journal*, **304**, 1127–8

Strang J & Gossop M (eds.) (1994). *Heroin Addiction and Drug Policy: The British System*. Oxford: Oxford University Press

Strang J & Sheridan J (1997a). Heroin prescribing in the 'British System' of the mid 1990s: data from the 1995 national survey of community pharmacies in England and Wales. *Drug and Alcohol Review*, **16**, 7–16

Strang J & Sheridan J (1997b). Prescribing amphetamines to drug misusers: Data from the 1995 National Survey of Community Pharmacies in England & Wales. *Addiction*, **92**, 833–8

Strang J, Donmall M, Webster A & Tantam D (1991). Comparison between community drug teams with and without inbuilt medical services. *British Medical Journal*, **303**, 897

Strang J, Smith M & Spurrell S (1992). The community drug team. *British Journal of Addiction*, **87**, 169–78

Strang J, Seivewright N & Farrell M (1993). Oral and intravenous abuse of benzodiazepines. In: Hallstrom C (ed.) *Benzodiazepine Dependence*. Oxford: Oxford Medical Publications, pp. 128–42

Strang J, Sheridan J & Barber N (1996). Prescribing injectable and oral methadone to opiate addicts: results from the 1995 national postal survey of community pharmacies in England and Wales. *British Medical Journal*, **313**, 270–2

Strang J, Marks I, Dawe S, Powell J, Gossop M, Richards D & Gray J (1997). Type of hospital setting and treatment outcome with heroin addicts. Results from a randomised trial. *British Journal of Psychiatry*, **171**, 335–9

Suffett F & Brotman R (1984). A comprehensive care program for pregnant addicts: obstetrical, neonatal and child development outcomes. *International Journal of Addictions*, **19**, 199–219

Swanson J, Holzer C & Ganju V (1990). Violence and psychiatric disorder in the community: evidence from the Epidemiological Catchment Area Survey. *Hospital and Community Psychiatry*, **41**, 761–70

Swofford CD, Kasckow JW, Scheller-Gilkey G & Inderbitzin LB (1996). Substance use: a powerful predictor of relapse in schizophrenia. *Schizophrenia Research*, **20**, 145–51

Tardiff K, Marzuk PM, Leon AC, Portera L, Hartwell N, Hirsch CS & Stajic M (1996). Accidental fatal drug overdoses in New York City: 1990–1992. *American Journal of Drug and Alcohol Abuse*, **22**, 135–46

Tetlow VA & Merrill J (1996). Rapid determination of amphetamine stereoisomer ratios in urine by gas chromatography–mass spectroscopy. *Annals of Clinical Biochemistry*, **33**, 50–4

Tretter F, Burkhardt D, Bussello-Spieth B, Reiss J, Walcher S & Buchele W (1998). Clinical experience with antagonist-induced opiate withdrawal under anaesthesia. *Addiction*, **93**, 269–75

Troisi A, Pasini A, Saracco M & Spalletta G (1998). Psychiatric symptoms in male cannabis users not using other illicit drugs. *Addiction*, **93**, 487–92

Tyrer P, Rutherford D & Huggett T (1981). Benzodiazepine withdrawal symptoms and propranolol. *Lancet*, **i**, 520–2

Tyrer P, Seivewright N, Ferguson B, Murphy S, Darling C, Brothwell J et al. (1990). The Nottingham Study of Neurotic Disorder: relationship between personality status and symptoms. *Psychological Medicine*, **20**, 423–31

Uchtenhagen A, Dobler-Mikola A & Gutzwiller (1996). Medical prescriptions of narcotics. *European Addiction Research*, **2**, 201–7

Vader JP & Aufseesser M (1993). Physicians and intravenous drug users: attitudes and opinions in the Canton of Vaud, Switzerland. *International Journal of the Addictions*, **28**, 1587–99

Verheul R, van den Brink W & Hartgers C (1995). Prevalence of personality disorders among alcoholics and drug addicts: an overview. *European Addiction Research*, **1**, 166–77

Wallace PG, Cutler S & Haines A (1988). Randomised controlled trial of general practitioner intervention in patients with excessive alcohol consumption. *British Medical Journal*, **297**, 663–8

Waller T & Holmes R (1995). Hepatitis C: scale and impact in Britain. *Druglink*, Sept/Oct, 8–11

Walsh SL, Preston KL, Stitzer ML, Cone EJ & Bigelow GE (1994). Clinical pharmacology of buprenorphine: ceiling effects at high doses. *Clinical Pharmacology and Therapeutics*, **55**, 569–80

Walsh SL, June HL, Schuh KJ, Preston KL, Bigelow GE & Stitzer ML (1995). Effects of buprenorphine in methadone-maintained subjects. *Psychopharmacology*, **119**, 268–76

Wanigaratne S, Wallis W, Pullin J, Keaney F & Farmer R (1990). *Relapse Prevention for Addictive Behaviours*. Oxford: Blackwell Scientific Publications

Ward J, Mattick RP & Hall W (1998a). The use of urinalysis during opioid replacement therapy. In: Ward J, Mattick RP & Hall W (eds.) *Methadone Maintenance Treatment and Other Opioid Replacement Therapies* London: Harwood, pp. 239–64

Ward J, Mattick RP & Hall W (1998b). How long is long enough? Answers to questions about the duration of methadone maintenance treatment. In: Ward J, Mattick RP & Hall W (eds.) *Methadone Maintenance Treatment and Other Opioid Replacement Therapies*. London: Harwood, pp. 305–36

Warner EA (1993). Cocaine abuse. *Annals of Internal Medicine*, **119**, 226

Warner EA, Kosten TR & O'Connor PG (1997). Pharmacotherapy for opioid and cocaine abuse. *Medical Clinics of North America*, **81**, 909–25

Washton AM & Resnick RB (1981). Clonidine in opiate withdrawal: review and appraisal of clinical findings. *Pharmacotherapy*, **1**, 140–6

Washton AM, Resnick RB & Geyer G (1983). Opiate withdrawal using lofexidine, a clonidine analogue with fewer side effects. *Journal of Clinical Psychiatry*, **44**, 335–7

Weddington WW, Brown BS, Haertzen CA, Cone EJ, Dax EM, Herning RI et al. (1990). Changes in mood, craving, and sleep during short-term abstinence reported by male cocaine addicts. *Archives in General Psychiatry*, **47**, 861–8

Wells P (1998). Hepatitis: the junkie disease. *Druglink*, Mar/Apr, 10–13

Westermeyer J (1995). Cultural aspects of substance abuse and alcoholism. *Psychiatric*

*Clinics of North America*, **18**, 589–605

White AP (1994). The promise, problems and limitations of methadone: a clinical perspective. *Journal of Clinical Forensic Medicine*, **1**, 97–140

Williams H, Oyefeso A & Ghodse AH (1996). Benzodiazepine misuse and dependence among opiate addicts in treatment. *Irish Journal of Psychological Medicine*, **13**, 62–4

Williamson S, Gossop M, Powis B, Griffiths, Foutain J & Strang J (1997). Adverse effects of stimulant drugs in a community sample of drug users. *Drug and Alcohol Dependence*, **44**, 87–94

Wilson GS, Desmond MM & Wait RB (1981). Follow-up of methadone-treated and untreated narcotic-dependent women and their infants: health, developmental and social implications. *Journal of Pediatrics*, **98**, 716–22

Withers NW, Pulvirenti L, Koob GF & Gillin JC (1995). Cocaine abuse and dependence. *Journal of Clinical Psychopharmacology*, **15**, 63–78

Wodak A (1994). Managing illicit drug use: a practical guide. *Drugs*, **47**, 446–57

Wodak A (1996). A stupendous public health achievement: commentary on Stimson's 'Has the United Kingdom averted an epidemic of HIV-1 infection among drug injectors?' *Addiction*, **91**, 1090–2

Wodak A (1997) . Hepatitis C: waiting for the Grim Reaper. *Medical Journal of Australia*, **166**, 290–3

Wodak A, Seivewright NA, Wells B, Reuter P, Des Jarlais DC, Rezza G, et al. (1994). Comments on: Ball & van de Wijngaart's 'A Dutch addict's view on methadone maintenance – an American and a Dutch appraisal'. *Addiction*, **89**, 803 14

Wolock I & Magura S (1996). Parental substance abuse as a predictor of child maltreatment. *Child Abuse and Neglect*, **20**, 1183–93

Wolstein J, Rosinger C & Gastpar M (1998). Children and families in substance misuse. *Current Opinion in Psychiatry*, **11**, 279–83

Wolters RDF (1995). Crime, disorder and legal pressure as a result of addiction problems in the Netherlands. *Medicine and Law*, **14**, 521–9

Woods JR (1996). Adverse consequences of prenatal illicit drug exposure. *Current Opinion in Obstetrics and Gynaecology*, **8**, 403–11

Worm K, Steentoft A & Kringsholm B (1993). Methadone and drug addicts. *International Journal of Legal Medicine*, **106**, 119–23

Wysowski DK, Schober SE, Wise RP & Kopstein A (1993). Mortality attributed to misuse of psychoactive drugs, 1979–88. *Public Health Reports*, **108**, 565–70

Yancovitz SR, Des Jarlais DC, Peyser NP, Drew E, Freidmann P, Trigg HL & Robinson JW (1991). A randomised trial of an interim methadone maintenance clinic. *American Journal of Public Health*, **81**, 1185–91

Zador D, Sunjic S & Darke S (1996). Heroin-related deaths in New South Wales, 1992: toxicological findings and circumstances. *Medical Journal of Australia*, **164**, 204–7

Ziedonis DM & Kosten TR (1991). Depression as a prognostic factor for pharmacological treatment of cocaine dependence. *Psychopharmacology Bulletin*, **27**, 337–43

Zweben JE (1986). Recovery-orientated psychotherapy. *Journal of Substance Abuse Treatment*, **3**, 255–62

# Index